Outpatient Plastic Surgery

Editors

GEOFFREY R. KEYES
ROBERT SINGER

CLINICS IN PLASTIC SURGERY

www.plasticsurgery.theclinics.com

July 2013 • Volume 40 • Number 3

ELSEVIER

1600 John F. Kennedy Boulevard ● Suite 1800 ● Philadelphia, Pennsylvania, 19103-2899

http://www.theclinics.com

CLINICS IN PLASTIC SURGERY Volume 40, Number 3
July 2013 ISSN 0094-1298, ISBN-13: 978-1-4557-7606-1

Editor: Joanne Husovski
Development Editor: Donald Mumford

Clinics in Plastic Surgery (ISSN 0094-1298) is published quarterly by Elsevier Inc., 360 Park Avenue South, New York, NY 10010-1710. Months of issue are January, April, July, and October. Business and Editorial Offices: 1600 John F. Kennedy Blvd., Suite 1800, Philadelphia, PA 19103-2899. Periodicals postage paid at New York, NY and additional mailing offices. Subscription prices are $466.00 per year for US individuals, $693.00 per year for US institutions, $229.00 per year for US students and residents, $529.00 per year for Canadian individuals, $809.00 per year for Canadian institutions, $607.00 per year for international individuals, $809.00 per year for international institutions, and $289.00 per year for Canadian and foreign students/residents. To receive student/resident rate, orders must be accompanied by name of affiliated institution, date of term, and the *signature* of program/residency coordinator on institution letterhead. Orders will be billed at individual rate until proof of status is received. Foreign air speed delivery is included in all *Clinics* subscription prices. All prices are subject to change without notice. **POSTMASTER:** Send address changes to *Clinics in Plastic Surgery*, Elsevier Health Sciences Division, Subscription Customer Service, 3251 Riverport Lane, Maryland Heights, MO 63043. **Customer Service: 1-800-654-2452 (US and Canada). From outside of the United States and Canada, call 314-447-8871. Fax: 314-447-8029. E-mail: JournalsCustomerService-usa@elsevier.com (for print support); JournalsOnlineSupport-usa@ elsevier.com (for online support).**

Reprints. For copies of 100 or more of articles in this publication, please contact the Commercial Reprints Department, Elsevier Inc., 360 Park Avenue South, New York, New York 10010-1710. Tel.: (+1) 212-633-3812; Fax: (+1) 212-462-1935; E-mail: reprints@elsevier.com.

Clinics in Plastic Surgery is covered in *Current Contents, EMBASE/Excerpta Medica, Science Citation Index, MEDLINE/ PubMed (Index Medicus), ASCA,* and *ISI/BIOMED.*

Printed and bound by CPI Group (UK) Ltd, Croydon, CR0 4YY

Transferred to digital print 2013

Contributors

EDITORS

GEOFFREY R. KEYES, MD, FACS
President – American Association for Accreditation of Ambulatory Surgery Facilities, Inc (AAAASF); Clinical Associate Professor of Plastic Surgery, Department of Plastic Surgery, Keck School of Medicine, University of Southern California, Los Angeles, California

ROBERT SINGER, MD, FACS
Clinical Professor Surgery (Plastic) - University of California, San Diego; Prior President, American Association for Accreditation of Ambulatory Surgery Facilities, Inc (AAAASF), La Jolla, California

AUTHORS

JEFFREY L. APFELBAUM, MD
Professor and Chairman, Department of Anesthesia and Critical Care, University of Chicago, Chicago, Illinois

PAMELA A. BAKER, CAE
Director of Surveyor Quality Assurance, AAAASF, Gurnee, Illinois

GARY M. BROWNSTEIN, MD
Member of AAAASF Board of Directors, Chairman, Quality Assurance Committee, AAAASF Private Practice, Plastic Surgery, Cherry Hill, New Jersey

THOMAS W. CUTTER, MD, MEd
Professor and Associate Chairman, Department of Anesthesia and Critical Care, University of Chicago, Chicago, Illinois

PETER B. FODOR, MD, FACS
Associate Clinical Professor, Plastic Surgery, UCLA Medical Center, Los Angeles, California

SUSAN FORMAN, CRNA
Allied Health Professional, Texas Institute for Surgery, Dallas, Texas

MICHAEL FRANK, MD
Clinical Associate Professor of Medicine, New York University School of Medicine, New York, New York; Attending Physician, Lenox Hill Hospital, New York, New York

ALAN GOLD, MD
Aesthetic Plastic Surgery & Cosmetic Medicine, Great Neck, NY

JANET L. GOMEZ, RN, BA, RNFA
R.N. First Assistant and Plastic Surgical Nurse/Skin Care Specialist, Ronald E. Iverson, MD, FACS, The Plastic Surgery Center, Pleasanton, California

MICHAEL HERNANDEZ, MD
Assistant Professor, Department of Anesthesia and Critical Care, University of Chicago Medicine, Chicago, Illinois

RONALD E. IVERSON, MD, FACS
Adjunct Clinical Professor of Plastic Surgery, Stanford University Medical School, Palo Alto, California; Member, Board of Directors, American Association for the Accreditation of Surgical Facilities, Illinois

TRIPTI KATARIA, MD
Assistant Professor, Department of Anesthesia and Critical Care, University of Chicago Medicine, Chicago, Illinois

GEOFFREY R. KEYES, MD, FACS
President – American Association for Accreditation of Ambulatory Surgery Facilities, Inc, (AAAASF); Clinical Associate Professor of Plastic Surgery, Department of Plastic Surgery, Keck School of Medicine, University of Southern California, Los Angeles, California

MARY KEYES, MD
Clinical Professor of Anesthesiology, UCLA
Department of Anesthesiology, Ronald
Reagan UCLA Medical Center, Los Angeles,
California

KATARZYNA LUBA, MD, MS
Assistant Professor, Department of Anesthesia
and Critical Care, University of Chicago,
Chicago, Illinois

MICHAEL F. MCGUIRE, MD, FACS
Clinical Professor, Division of Plastic Surgery,
Department of Surgery, University of Southern
California Los Angeles, California; Associate
Clinical Professor, Division of Plastic Surgery,
Department of Surgery, University
of California, Los Angeles, Los Angeles,
California

FOAD NAHAI, MD, FACS
Associate Professor of Plastic Surgery,
Emory University School of Medicine, Atlanta,
Georgia

SHEILA S. NAZARIAN MOBIN, MD, MMM
Resident Physician, Division of Plastic Surgery,
Keck School of Medicine of USC, Los Angeles,
California

JOHN D. NEWKIRK, PhD, MD
Plastic Surgeon, Private Practice, West
Columbia, Columbia, South Carolina

JEFF PEARCY, MPA, CAE
Executive Director, AAAASF, Gurnee, Illinois

HARLAN POLLOCK, MD
Clinical Instructor, Department of Plastic
Surgery, U.T. Southwestern Medical School;
Medical Staff, Texas Institute for Surgery;
T.H.R. Presbyterian Hospital of Dallas, Dallas,
Texas

TODD POLLOCK, MD
Clinical Instructor, Department of Plastic
Surgery, U.T. Southwestern Medical School;

Medical Staff, Texas Institute for Surgery;
T.H.R. Presbyterian Hospital of Dallas, Dallas,
Texas

MARK RACCASI, MD
Medical Staff, Texas Institute for Surgery;
T.H.R. Presbyterian Hospital of Dallas, Dallas,
Texas

LAWRENCE S. REED, MD, FACS
Assistant Professor of Surgery, The Weill
Cornell Medical Center, New York Presbytarian
Hospital, New York

ROBERT SINGER, MD, FACS
Clinical Professor Surgery (Plastic) - University
of California, San Diego; Prior President,
American Association for Accreditation of
Ambulatory Surgery Facilities, Inc (AAAASF),
La Jolla, California

ALI M. SOLTANI, MD
Hand Surgery Fellow, Division of Plastic,
Reconstructive and Aesthetic Surgery,
University of Miami/Jackson Memorial
Hospital, Miami, Florida

THOMAS TERRANOVA, MA
Director of External Relations, The American
Association for Accreditation of Ambulatory
Surgery Facilities, Inc, Gurnee, Illinois

DENNIS THOMPSON, MD, FACS
Clinical Professor of Plastic Surgery,
Department of Plastic Surgery, University
of California, Los Angeles, California

JAMES YATES, MD
Medical Director, Plastic & Cosmetic Surgery
Center, Camp Hill, Pennsylvania; Medical
Director, Grandview Surgery & Laser Center,
Camp Hill, Pennsylvania; Chief of Plastic
Surgery, Holy Spirit Hospital, Camp Hill,
Pennsylvania; Plastic Surgery Department,
Pinnacle Health System, Harrisburg,
Pennsylvania; Former President, AAAASF,
Gurnee, Illinois

Contents

Patient safety is the mission of the American Association for Accreditation of Ambulatory Surgery Facilities, Inc (AAAASF). Well-crafted standards are at the foundation of attaining successful Ambulatory Surgical Facility outcomes. Without expert inspection practices and administrative processes supporting these standards, they are powerless to protect patients. This 2-part approach is used by AAAASF to ensure 100% compliance of all surgical standards.

Ambulatory surgery is commonplace for a multitude of procedures and a wide range of patients. The types of procedures performed in the ambulatory setting are becoming more work-intensive, and patients with comorbidities make for a challenging environment. For a safe environment for surgery in ambulatory facilities, the complex task of patient selection is necessary. Until an algorithm is created that includes provider, procedure, facility, and patient comorbidites, clinicians must rely on general guidelines rather than precise recommendations.

The safety, efficacy, and rapid recovery of conscious sedation/local anesthesia make this anesthetic technique useful in the ambulatory setting. The care of the sedated patient requires a team effort. The individual role and responsibility of patient, surgeon, anesthesia provider, and nursing staff are discussed. Using data obtained from a series of 1400 consecutive cases, the authors' experience with conscious sedation/local anesthesia is presented. The current technique, using low-dose propofol, is described in detail. Using conscious sedation, the patient's level of consciousness is depressed, but respiratory drive and airway reflexes are maintained and anesthesia is provided by infiltration of local anesthetic.

This article summarizes current information on the risk and the assessment of risks for deep venous thrombosis (DVT) resulting from plastic surgery procedures. Risk assessment is the foundation for recommended methods of prevention of DVT and, in turn, possible pulmonary emboli. If prevention fails, treatment of DVT is required to avoid the major complication of pulmonary emboli. The significant risk of DVT and pulmonary emboli after an abdominoplasty is confirmed in this article.

Facilities–accredited facilities prove the contrary. There is a lack of data investigating infection prevention in the perioperative period in plastic surgery patients. As data collection becomes more refined, tracking the postoperative care environment should offer additional opportunities to lower the incidence of postoperative infections.

CLINICS IN PLASTIC SURGERY

Preface
Ambulatory Plastic Surgery: High Standards Set by Plastic Surgeons

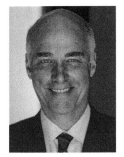 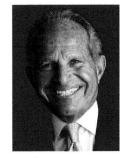

Geoffrey R. Keyes, MD   Robert Singer, MD

Editors

Ambulatory surgery facilities have increased in number dramatically over the past 50 years. Recognizing the need for safe, affordable, and accessible care, plastic surgeons had the vision to create the American Association for Accreditation of Ambulatory Surgery Facilities, Inc (AAAASF) in 1980.

The mandate for AAAASF was to create an accreditation program that would develop reasonable standards and improve the quality of medical and surgical care in ambulatory surgery facilities, assuring the public access to the best available care safety in accredited facilities.

In 1996, California became the first state to mandate accreditation for all outpatient facilities that administer sedation or general anesthesia. AAAASF was instrumental in the development of the California legislation (AB 595) as well as subsequent laws and regulations in Florida, Georgia, New Jersey, Pennsylvania, Texas, and many other states. AAAASF accreditation has been approved by some State Departments of Health in lieu of State Licensure and is a deemed authority for Medicare accreditation. Although AAAASF was initially developed by plastic surgeons for plastic surgical facilities, the preponderance of AAAASF's accredited facilities are now in specialties other than plastic surgery.

Accrediting more than 2000 ambulatory facilities, including office-based, free-standing surgical centers that are used by one or multispecialties, AAAASF has taken a leadership role in championing the need for all states to require accreditation or licensure for all outpatient facilities.

AAAASF has led the way in data collection to improve patient care through the development of an Internet-based Quality Assurance Program that has collected over 9,000,000 procedures for analysis. Currently, AAAASF is innovating new methods of data collection to foster the practice of surgery through evidence-based medicine and to raise the bar of safety for the public and the surgeons operating in these facilities.

This *Clinics in Plastic Surgery* publication focuses on outpatient surgery, highlighting important information about safe surgical practice, and

Clin Plastic Surg 40 (2013) xi–xii
http://dx.doi.org/10.1016/j.cps.2013.06.001
0094-1298/13/$ – see front matter © 2013 Published by Elsevier Inc.

documents the excellent track record achieved by facilities accredited by AAAASF.

Geoffrey R. Keyes, MD
American Association for Accreditation of
Ambulatory Surgery Facilities, Inc
PO Box 95005101 Washington Street
2F Gurnee, IL 60031, USA
Department of Plastic Surgery
Keck School of Medicine
University of Southern California
Los Angeles, CA, USA
www.keycare.com

Robert Singer, MD
American Association for Accreditation of
Ambulatory Surgery Facilities, Inc
PO Box 95005101 Washington Street
2F Gurnee, IL 60031, USA
University of California San Diego
La Jolla, CA, USA
www.rsingermd.com

E-mail addresses:
geoffkeyes@gmail.com (G.R. Keyes)
rsingermd@aol.com (R. Singer)

Outpatient Facility Standards
What is Necessary for Satisfactory Outcomes?

Gary M. Brownstein, MD[a],*, Pamela A. Baker, CAE[b]

KEYWORDS

- Patient safety • Standards composition and oversight • Educational training • Quality assurance
- Inspectors • Facilities

KEY POINTS

- Patient safety is the mission of the American Association for Accreditation of Ambulatory Surgery Facilities, Inc (AAAASF).
- Well-crafted standards are at the foundation of attaining successful standards outcomes.
- Without expert inspection practices and administrative processes supporting these standards, they are powerless to protect patients.
- This 2 part approach is used by AAAASF to ensure 100% compliance of all surgical standards.

PART 1: SURGICAL ENVIRONMENT
Stratification of Facilities Based on Administered Anesthesia

Facilities are often classified on the level of the anesthetic care offered. One classification would stratify the facilities as: Class 1, Local, Regional and Topical Anesthesia; Class 2, Parenteral Sedation (not including propofol); Class 3, Parenteral Sedation Including Propofol; and Class 4, General Anesthesia. In the case of Class 3 and Class 4, an anesthesiologist or certified registered nurse anesthetist (CRNA) would be required to administer the anesthetic.

In Class 2, a qualified physician could supervise the administration of a parenteral sedation.[1]

Operating Suite (Physical Plant)

An operating suite should include an operating room (OR), scrub area, clean area, dirty area, and a recovery room. The operating suite needs to be physically separate from the general office.

The OR should be a separate and distinct area in the suite, dedicated specifically for surgical use.

All major surgery is to be performed in the OR. To maintain the sterile atmosphere, unauthorized individuals should be deterred from entering the OR. The OR should be adequately ventilated and temperature controlled for safety reasons. Hypothermia is known to increase risk of arrhythmias and infection.

The available square footage in the OR must be adequate to hold all of the personnel, equipment, sterile supplies, and medications necessary to perform the surgical procedure. It should be sufficient to accommodate emergency situations and the personnel necessary to evacuate a patient in the case of an unforeseen event. Efficiency and sterility dictate that personnel leaving the operating room to obtain supplies should be kept to a minimum, and that the storage space in the OR should allow for easy identification and inventory of the supplies.

Surfaces in the OR, such as the countertops, ceiling surface, and floors, should be smooth, easily washable, and free of particular material that might cause contamination. There must not be any tears, breaks, or cracks in these surfaces that could

[a] Quality Assurance Committee, AAAASF Private Practice, Plastic Surgery, Cherry Hill, NJ, USA; [b] AAAASF, P.O. Box 9500, Gurnee, IL 60031, USA
* Corresponding author.
E-mail addresses: gbrownstein@comcast.net; pamela@aaaasf.org

Clin Plastic Surg 40 (2013) 363–370
http://dx.doi.org/10.1016/j.cps.2013.04.001
0094-1298/13/$ – see front matter © 2013 Published by Elsevier Inc.

harbor bacteria. Any seams should be sealed with an impermeable sealant other than silicone.

The recovery-area space allocated in the suite should be sufficient to accommodate the necessary personnel, equipment, and monitoring devices necessary for a safe recovery. This area needs to be stocked with readily accessible equipment and medications for routine recoveries, as well as emergencies. Similar to the OR, the postanesthesia care unit (PACU) should be easy to clean and free from fire hazards. Space available for sterilizing instruments should be segregated into a dirty area where contaminated instruments are cleaned, and a clean area for packaging and sterilization. Separation between dirty and clean areas may be accomplished by a wall, distance, or time. The same area may be used for both purposes if, and only if, it is the documented policy of the facility to clean and disinfect the dirty utility area before assembly of packages for sterilization occurs.

Fire in an operating suite can be disastrous. Proper preparation and avoidance of problems may mitigate the devastating effects including injury and loss of life. The facility must be equipped with heat sensors and/or smoke detectors and an adequate number of appropriately placed fire extinguishers that are inspected annually. Fire-exit signs are posted and adequate emergency lighting is available. A smoke-filled room can become dark very quickly, and appropriate lighting is critical. All safety regulations of the Occupational Safety and Health Administration (OSHA) should be followed to help decrease the risk of fire. Appropriate fire precautions must be in place when using a cautery or a laser during the administration of oxygen.

Fire safety mandates that the operating suite contain sufficient number of electrical outlets that are labeled and grounded. There must be a source of emergency power, such as a generator or battery-powered inverter, with the capacity to operate anesthesia, surgical equipment, and lighting for an amount of time that is consistent with procedures performed. The generated power should be available seamlessly within 30 seconds of the power failure. Pertinent safeguards require that essential equipment should be connected to the emergency power source during surgery and recovery, thus preventing a situation whereby personnel are frantically looking for backup power outlets during an outage or, worse, in a smoke-filled room. The backup power equipment should be checked on a monthly basis and a log kept of the checks.

Equipment

Boxes 1–3 list the basic equipment that should be contained in the operating room and PACU. The

---

> **Box 1**
> **Operating room equipment**
>
> 1. Adequate washable operating room table or chair
> 2. Adequate ceiling lighting
> 3. Electrocardiography monitor with pulse read-out
> 4. Pulse oximeter
> 5. Blood pressure monitoring equipment
> 6. Standard defibrillator, or an automated external defibrillator unit
> 7. Sequential compressive devices
> 8. Electrocautery with a grounding plate or disposable pad

equipment requirement may vary somewhat depending on the type of anesthesia administered in the facility.

The specifications, that is, the manufacturer's recommendations for the equipment's operation, maintenance, and cleaning, should be kept in an organized file available to all staff. Safety standards demand that only inspected equipment is permitted to be used in the suite. All equipment should be inspected at least annually by a biomedical technician. Detailed records of the equipment inspections should be kept. Some equipment, such as sterilizers, should be checked weekly with spore tests or an equivalent, and the records maintained. Automated external defibrillators and

---

> **Box 2**
> **Anesthesia equipment**
>
> 1. Laryngoscope
> 2. Appropriately sized oral airways, nasopharyngeal airways, and laryngeal mask airways
> 3. Endotracheal tubes
> 4. Endotracheal stylet
> 5. Positive pressure ventilation device (eg, Ambu bag)
> 6. Source of O_2
> 7. Source of suction
> 8. CO_2 monitor
> 9. Anesthesia machine
>   i. Mechanical ventilator with disconnect device
>   ii. Purge system
>   iii. Inspired gas oxygen monitor

Box 3 Recovery room equipment
1. A reliable source and amount of oxygen, regulators, tubing, and masks 2. Adequate and reliable source of suction 3. Self-inflating (Ambu) bags, capable of delivering positive pressure ventilation with at least 90% oxygen concentration 4. Adequate illumination for patients, machines, and monitoring equipment 5. Sufficient available electrical outlets, labeled and grounded to suit the equipment and connected to emergency power supplies where appropriate 6. Emergency cart available with defibrillator, necessary drugs, and other cardiopulmonary resuscitation equipment 7. Separate pulse oximeter available for each patient

defibrillators should also be checked weekly and a performance log kept. Any repairs should be performed and documented by a biomedical technician.

Instrument Sterilization

The facility is required to have at least one autoclave that uses high-pressure steam. A gas sterilizer is an acceptable addition, and must be vented properly. High-level disinfectants, such as Cidex, may only be used for nonautoclavable equipment by which contact will be made with mucous membranes or other body surfaces that are not sterile. Protocols for proper handling and sterilization of equipment should be present in the Policy and Procedure manual (for an example of a high-level disinfection protocol, see **Box 4**).[2] If the sterilizer produces monitoring records, they should be logged. If no monitoring record is produced, best practices may include production of a sterilizing log noting each load that is sterilized by whom, the date, the cycle that it was sterilized on, and so forth.

Storage of sterile supplies should be away from potentially contaminated areas; sterile packages should be labeled to indicate date of sterilization and, if necessary, when the sterility should expire. Sterile supplies should be packaged and sealed to prevent accidental opening and, if more than 1 sterilizer is available in the facility, the package should be labeled as to which sterilizer was used, in the case of a positive spore test. Sterile and clean supplies should not be stored in the

Box 4 Processing an endoscope
• The location of the manual rinsing and cleaning of endoscopes before high-level disinfection may be performed in the procedure room away from the patient • Specific steps must be in place to minimize spraying and aerosolizing of the bio-burden • Processing of the scopes must be in the location that meets requisite standards of air exchange ratios and vapor particle standards • Necessary protective equipment for personnel must be available • Scope-cleaning functions should be limited to properly trained personnel • If there is not a separate room (see previous standard) being used for processing of the scopes, the protocol must include steps directing that the contaminated equipment will be cleaned and placed in the reprocessor before bringing the next patient into the room. In addition, the clean scope coming out of the reprocessor is to be removed only when the room is clean and free of dirty instruments • Cross-contamination should be avoided no matter where cleaning and processing takes place. There must always be some distinct type of separation of clean and dirty areas in any location • Clean (reprocessed) endoscopes should be stored in a closed cabinet exclusively dedicated to scope storage, to avoid contamination before use • High-level disinfection is used only for nonautoclavable endoscopic equipment, and in areas that are categorized as semicritical where contact will be made with mucous membrane or other body surfaces that are not sterile • At all times the manufacturer's recommendations for use should be followed

same space. Sterile packages should not be stored above a steam autoclave, to prevent contamination.

Cleaning the Facility

The entire operating suite should be cleaned and disinfected according to an established schedule created specifically to prevent cross-contamination. Blood and body-fluid spills are cleaned using an intermediate-level disinfectant (sporicidal, bactericidal, fungicidal, and virucidal).

If the cleaning personnel are not part of the staff, they should sign a HIPAA (Health Insurance Portability and Accountability Act 1996) compliant confidentiality agreement in the event that any patient information is visible.

Medical wastes are stored in OSHA-acceptable containers and separated for special collection. Disposable sharps are kept in a puncture-resistant container close to the area where they are used. Finally, all garments, scrub suits, linen, blankets, and so forth do not leave the facility to be washed at home, but are cleaned by an OSHA-compliant laundry; or, if the laundry is processed on premises, a protocol geared to rid the laundry of pathogens is followed.

Medication, Intravenous Fluids, Gases

All medications present must be in date and readily identifiable. It is critical that all personnel know the location of medications, especially emergency medications. An emergency cart with a defibrillator, necessary drugs, other cardiopulmonary resuscitation equipment (such as a source of suction and intravenous setup), and the Advanced Cardiopulmonary Life Support (ACLS) algorithms resides in the suite.

All controlled substances are to be secured and locked under supervised access. A bound or secured-computer narcotic inventory and control record is required. This record must be dated and include the patient's name or ID number, and be verified by 2 licensed members of the OR team at least weekly as well as on the day any of these agents are administered.

It is required that intravenous fluid is present in every facility, even if just local or topical anesthetics are used. If the facility presents an unusual situation in having a means to obtain and administer, there must be a protocol for the blood to be typed, cross-matched, checked, and verified. Dextran, a blood substitute, should be present in the facility, or the facility should have a means of obtaining it on a timely basis.

If potential triggering agents are present in the facility, an appropriate malignant hyperthermia emergency protocol and setup must be available. Even if succinylcholine is present and is only to be used in dire circumstances such as for bronchospasm, this setup is required. An alternative to the drug of choice (succinylcholine) is the nondepolarizing and nontriggering agent, rocuronium.

A reliable source and amount of oxygen should be present, and must include a regulator as well as the tubing and mask. Other essential equipment for a facility that would be Class 2 or greater (see later discussion) would include a laryngeal mask airway or endotracheal tube necessary to deliver the oxygen. A self-inflating Ambu bag capable of delivering positive pressure ventilation with 90% oxygen concentration, and a separate pulse oximeter for each patient, are essential.

All explosive and combustible materials are stored and handled in a safe manner according to state, local, and/or National Fire Protection Association codes. Compressed-gas cylinders should be chained to the wall or placed in an appropriate carrier.

OR Suite Staff: Medical Director, Practitioners, Personnel

A Medical Director, specifically a physician (MD or DO), is a necessity. The Medical Director must actively participate in the management of the facility. The Medical Director must be currently licensed in the state where the facility is located. The team should include a nurse and anesthesiologist or CRNA when dissociative anesthesia, intravenous sedation with propofol, or general anesthesia is performed. Determining who is appropriately credentialed and qualified to perform procedures in the facility is an arduous task, as any physician who has obtained hospital privileges can attest. The required steps are practically impossible for a smaller facility to accomplish. Each facility cannot have its own criteria for credentialing. One solution to the credentialing dilemma is to require the practitioner be credentialed by an acute care hospital for privileges consistent with privileges requested of the facility.

In addition, following the American Medical Association core principle #7, it is essential that every individual who performs procedures in the facility needs to be "…currently board certified/qualified by one of the boards recognized by the American Board of Medical specialties, American Osteopathic Association, or a board with equivalent standards approved by the state medical board."[3] The procedures that the practitioner performs must be "generally recognized by that certifying board as falling within the scope of training and practice of the physician providing the care."[3] Appropriate board certification of podiatrists or oral surgeons must also be required.

The proof of acceptable credentials is evidenced by the practitioner's demonstration that he or she holds or has held unrestricted core privileges in his or her specialty at a licensed care hospital. The loss of hospital privileges may not be caused by a lack of clinical competence, ethical issues, and so forth; rather, the only acceptable reason for the loss of hospital privileges is economic credentialing by the care facility. If the practitioner has not maintained privileges, arrangements must be in place assuring that another practitioner of the same specialty with privileges at the local acute care hospital will assume care of the patient in the event of unforeseen hospital transfer of the patient.

Continued maintenance of privileges requires that each physician, podiatrist, or oral and maxillofacial surgeon submits to the facility a copy of his or her current appropriate state license. Any actions affecting the practitioner, Medical Director, or any other member of the team must be reported to the governing body within a reasonable specified time period.

The personnel who work in the OR suite must meet acceptable standards as defined by their professional governing bodies, where applicable. Every employee should have a file that contains documentation (as outlined in **Box 5**). Be aware that according to OSHA regulations, these files should be kept for 30 years. There should be a written manual containing job descriptions, confidentiality policies, vacation policies, payment procedures, and so forth. Every employee should become familiar with the policies contained in this manual.

There is a regularly employed and licensed registered nurse, physician (other than the operating surgeon), or physician's assistant designated as the person responsible for patient care in all areas of the suite. All operating suite personnel are under the immediate supervision of this individual.

The OR personnel must be knowledgable in treating cardiopulmonary and anaphylactic emergencies. The OR personnel are familiar with operation and location of equipment, medication, and procedures used in the treatment of such emergencies. At least one member of the OR team, preferably the surgeon or the anesthesia provider, must hold current ACLS certification. Everyone else should possess at least a current Basic Cardiopulmonary Life Support certification (see **Box 4**).

The safety of all OR suite personnel is essential. There is a written policy for personal protective equipment for specific tasks in the facility such as instrument cleaning, disposal of biological waste, and surgery. Badge testing is required if a gas sterilizer, x-ray equipment, or high-level disinfectant is used in the facility. A Facility Safety Manual should provide employees with information about hazardous chemicals used and methods to minimize exposure to them. Material safety data sheets on all potentially hazardous substances found in the facility should be located in this manual.

Anesthesia: Anesthesiologist/CRNA

In facilities where dissociative anesthesia with propofol, spinal or epidural blocks, or general anesthesia is administered, an anesthesiologist or CRNA must provide the anesthetic care. These individuals must be qualified for such patient care, their credentials verified, and the documentation kept on file. These persons must be responsible for the monitoring of all life-support systems and ensure that all anesthesia equipment is in proper working order.

If responsible for supervising anesthesia or providing anesthesia, the qualified physician or CRNA must be present in the operating suite throughout the anesthetic. If sedation is being supervised by the operating surgeon, he or she must have knowledge of anesthetics and resuscitative techniques. Podiatrists and oral surgeons must use an anesthesiologist or a supervising physician to administer anesthesia other than local.

A physician is responsible for determining the medical status of the patient, and must examine the patient immediately before surgery. The anesthesia care provider must verify that an anesthesia care plan has been developed and documented. The patient must be informed of such a plan and receive preoperative instruction by the anesthesia provider supervising the anesthetic.

Box 5
Required personnel documentation

- Personnel records should contain:
  - Resumé of training and experience
  - Current certification or license if required by the state
  - Date of employment
  - Description of duties
  - Record of continuing education
  - Inoculations or refusals
- Proof of training:
  - Hazard safety training
  - Blood-borne pathogens
  - Universal precautions
  - Other safety training such as operation of a fire extinguisher
  - At least Basic Cardiopulmonary Life Support certification, or Advanced Cardiac Life Support (ACLS)
  - ACLS for one member in each operating room and recovery room team is required

During the procedure, besides administering medication the individual responsible for the anesthetic care should monitor and record the patient's vital signs on a frequent basis. Appropriate fluids should be administered, oxygenation maintained, and temperature monitored, especially if clinically significant changes in body temperature are expected. Forced air warmers, blanket warmers, or other devices should be used to maintain patient temperature. Sequential compression devices should be used for cases other than local anesthesia and of longer duration.

Anesthesia personnel should be familiar with the facility's emergency protocol for cardiopulmonary emergencies and other internal and external disasters. These individuals should be trained and knowledgable about the facility's protocols for safe and timely transfer of a patient to an alternative care facility when extended or emergency services are required.

Protocols, Policies, and Procedures

PACU

After the procedure is completed the patient is transferred to the PACU, where he or she will recover from the anesthetic. During this monitored trip the patient needs to be accompanied by a member of the anesthesia team who is knowledgable about the patient's condition. It will be necessary for the accompanying staff to provide the necessary information to the PACU personnel. The patient is evaluated in the PACU, and vital functions are supported as needed until the patient stabilizes. Initially, recovery room staff must evaluate the patient and record a set of vital signs. Observation and monitoring in the PACU must be by methods appropriate to the patient's condition and include ventilation, circulation, temperature, and mentation. A physician, CRNA, physician assistant, or registered nurse should directly supervise the recovery room care. The responsible individual must be currently licensed by the appropriate state, certified in ACLS, and immediately available until the patient has left the PACU.

The course of events in the PACU, similar to that in the OR, needs to be documented, starting with the patient's time of arrival. The recovery-room record should reflect the recovery course with entries of medications given to the patient, nursing notes, vital signs, and fluid administration.

For discharge from the PACU to occur, approved and standardized criteria need to be met. The determination that discharge criteria have been achieved must be performed and documented by a physician, based on input from the PACU personnel. Written instructions including procedures for emergency situations must be given to an adult who is responsible for the patient's care and transportation and to the patient. Personnel will assist in discharging the patient from the PACU, accomplished by wheelchair or gurney as needed.

Other policies and protocols

Plans of action should be in place for the following: cardiopulmonary resuscitation; malignant hyperthermia; security emergencies such as an intruder in the facility; an unruly patient or visitor; a threat to the staff or patients; fire; unplanned return to the operating room; a surgeon, anesthesiologist, or CRNA becoming incapacitated; and power-failure emergencies. Best practices would also include a deep vein thrombosis/emboli protocol.

Drills

The purpose of a drill is to convert a set of actions into a coherent plan that is practiced, so that when and if an emergent or threatening event occurs appropriate action ensues, rather than chaos. The tasks required should be detailed with regard to the specific action required, how to accomplish the task, and which team member should be assigned to perform the task. Drills should include, but not be limited to, fire drills, emergency evacuation of the facility, and malignant hyperthermia and cardiopulmonary resuscitation.

Patient's bill of rights

A copy of the patient's rights is prominently displayed, or a copy is provided to each patient. It is important that the Bill of Rights is adhered to by all facility personnel.

Documentation: Medical Records

Medical records are to be kept in the facility. The record should include an intake sheet completed by the patient providing most of his or her medical history and demographics. A history and physical examination commensurate with the procedure to be performed, a preoperative anesthesia evaluation with an anesthesia care plan, and informed consent should be contained in the chart. All laboratory results must be present and reviewed. The review should be initialed and dated by the surgeon at the time of evaluation. All other reports, such as pathology reports and medical clearance reports, must be reviewed and initialed. A written operative report, anesthesia record, and recovery record should be present. Best practice would also include an OR record. Finally, postoperative notes should be present.

Quality Assessment and Quality Improvement

The facility has a written quality improvement program in place, which should include surveys of projects that monitor and evaluate patient care, evaluate methods to improve patient care, identify and correct deficiencies within the facility, and alert the Medical Director to identify and resolve problems. To monitor performance, a review of a set number of random cases and any operative sequelae occurring within 30 days of the surgery should be performed on a regular basis. Peer review must be conducted by a recognized peer-review organization or a physician, podiatrist, or oral and maxillofacial surgeon other than the operating surgeon.

Each Unanticipated Operative Sequelae chart review must include the following information, in addition to the operation performed: identification of the problem, immediate treatment or disposition of the case, outcome, reason for problem, and assessment of efficacy of treatment.

PART 2: MAINTENANCE AND OVERSIGHT
Maintenance of Standards

The first part of this article describes the necessary components of the surgical environment required to produce safe outcomes. The mechanism of regulating such environmental necessities is best accomplished by the generation of a set of standards that precisely and concisely describe these requirements. Compliance with these standards engenders safety, and the facility's sustained adherence to the requirements is essential to continued success. In addition, following these standards must allow for the creation of a facility that has the potential for safe outcomes.

Accrediting Organization

To ensure the provision, implementation, and maintenance of the standard, an independent organization is required, whose purpose is to provide accreditation to facilities that are in compliance. The test for compliance is an inspection. The methods used to implement standards should be predominantly educational.

The accrediting organization should have a national recognized presence and reputation for excellence in medical and surgical standards, along with the substantial, dedicated resources to support the necessary high level of service and trained management for the standards programs. A well-trained accreditation staff must be available to process the application and inspection phases of new and renewed facilities. In addition, systems and equipment must be upgraded and ready to store mandatory accreditation documents for annual reference by accreditation staff. Inquiries from state medical boards, national regulatory organizations, and law firms require the ability to provide expedited and accurate responses from the accreditation staff concerning accredited facilities.

Oversight of all of the processes and final decisions ultimately resides with the Board of Directors. This board comprises surgeons, anesthesiologists, CRNAs, nurses, and public members.

Standards

To be functional, there are many characteristics that the standards should possess. Standards must be clear and concise. Every individual reading the standard should derive the same meaning or intent from the standard. There should not be any room for interpretation. Each standard should be objective. To alleviate subjectivity requires that each standard should have "yes" or "no" answers with respect to compliance. Every standard should be specific, addressing a single attribute of the environment.

A committee of individuals who possess significant awareness of surgical processes should be charged to provide the standards' content. The composition of this body should be predominantly surgical clinicians. This committee should meet regularly to review all standards in a rotational framework to ensure all medical standards have received supervision to stay current with clinical standards of practice, equipment, medication improvements, and safety.

Input into the committee should come from many sources. Many of the standards require a perusal of other organizations that produce successful outcomes, such as hospitals. The object of outpatient care is to reduce the cumbersome or nonessential elements to provide a limited scope of care. The committee should work closely with regulatory organizations such as OSHA, the Centers for Disease Control and Prevention, HIPAA, the Association of Perioperative Registered Nurses, and other similar national authorities, along with medical specialty associations, to stay current on new procedures, updates in standards of practice, and alerts on patient safety.

The Inspection

The test for measuring a facility's compliance with the standards is the inspection. In the authors' experience, surgeons seem to make the best examiners. Of course, for larger facilities a team of inspectors is necessary. The team is significantly benefited by nurses and anesthesiologists. The level of surgical sophistication is high, and helps provide standardization. It is almost comforting to the facility's Medical Director to know that he or she will be dealing with another physician who can manifest a clear understanding of the standards. Despite their background, inspectors will be required to undergo training by the accreditation organization, which may be accomplished through various methods including seminars, webinars, DVDs, and newsletters.

The inspection is, in essence, an "open book test." The standards book is presented to each facility ahead of time. There must not be any confusion over what is necessary and what will be examined. The process of the inspection involves the inspector to read and test each standard. For example, if the standard calls for a policy for a "time-out," the inspector will request to see the written policy requiring a time-out including the content of the time-out. There is the potential that a certain standard may not be applicable to a specific facility. The fact that it does not apply would require that a reason be specified.

After inspection, a list of deficiencies is provided to the facility. Any deficiency found must be rectified within 30 days of the reported inspection. It must be understood that a deficiency left uncorrected could result in decertification.

Oversight of the inspectors is the work of the Quality Assurance committee. Data are collected on all inspectors with the goal of using the data to improve the inspector pool. It is the goal of the entire organization to generate standardization, so that any inspection done by any inspector in any location would yield the same results.

Validation of Standards

A program of reported and collected peer-review information is critical in keeping abreast of patient safety issues and trends. It is required that all facilities submit peer review, including a random review of record and operative sequelae, at least biannually to maintain accreditation. Some sequelae need to be reported more quickly; for example, an operative death must be reported within 5 days of the knowledge of its occurrence.

An organization that requires the timely reporting of unanticipated sequelae is supporting definitive patient safety evidence on behalf of the accredited facilities and their surgical specialties. Accrediting organizations collect patient safety data based on their standards. These collected statistics are then able to validate that facilities' safety rates are acceptable.

Evidence-based medicine has entered into consideration with the development of medical standards providing up-to-date and precise content for the oversight of all standards. A future vision would be to generate data through AAAAF's Internet-Based Quality Assurance and Peer-Review Program (IBQUA) which, by virtue of its large sample size, has the potential to provide better evidence for delivery of safe surgical care through the integration of perioperative care data points with outcomes.[4,5]

SUMMARY

Patient safety should remain at the core of all successful outpatient standards, now and into the future. Quantified surgical safety data, along with the development of new and safer surgical procedures, are combining to create safe surgical standards for the benefit of all. More than 2000 years ago Cicero said: "The safety of the people is the supreme law [salus populi suprema lex]."

REFERENCES

1. AAAASF regular surgical standards, version 13. Available at: http://www.ironworks.us.com/asfall/PDFs%20Common/ASF%20ASC%20Standards%20and%20Checklist%20-%20Regular.pdf. Accessed November 2012.
2. AAAASF procedural standards, version 3. Available at: http://www.ironworks.us.com/asfall/PDFs%20Common/PROC%20Standards%20and%20Checklist%20-%20Procedural.pdf. Accessed November 2012.
3. Office based surgery core principles, principal #7. Available at: http://www.ama-assn.org/ama1/pub/upload/mm/370/obscoreprinciples.pdf. Accessed November 2012.
4. Keyes GR, Singer R, Iverson RE, et al. Analysis of outpatient surgery center safety using an internet-based quality improvement and peer review program. Plast Reconstr Surg 2004;113(6):1760–70.
5. Keyes GR, Singer R, Iverson RE, et al. Mortality in outpatient surgery. Plast Reconstr Surg 2008; 122(1):245–50.

Patient Selection in Outpatient Surgery

Tripti Kataria, MD, Thomas W. Cutter, MD, MEd,
Jeffrey L. Apfelbaum, MD*

KEYWORDS

- Outpatient surgery • Obesity • Cardiovascular disease • Pulmonary risk factors • Elderly patients
- Diabetes mellitus

KEY POINTS

- Ambulatory surgery is commonplace for a multitude of procedures and a wide range of patients.
- The types of procedures performed in the ambulatory setting are becoming more work-intensive, and patients with comorbidities make for a challenging environment.
- For a safe environment for surgery in ambulatory facilities, the complex task of patient selection is necessary.
- Until an algorithm is created that includes provider, procedure, facility, and patient comorbidities, clinicians rely on general guidlines rather than precise recommendations.
- When determining if a patient is suitable for ambulatory surgery, multiple factors must be assessed.

Ambulatory surgical volume in the United States increased 300% between 1992 and 2006.[1,2] In 2006, an estimated 53.3 million procedures were performed in ambulatory centers, 19.9 million in hospitals, and 14.9 million in freestanding surgical centers.[2] The increase has occurred partly because of financial incentives, changes in clinical practice from advances in technology, and patient expectations. Whether a case is appropriate for the ambulatory setting depends on where the surgery will occur, the personnel involved, the surgical procedure, and the patient's medical status. Consideration of these 4 criteria will help achieve optimal patient outcomes.

Ambulatory surgery can occur in a physician's office, freestanding ambulatory surgical center, building on a medical campus, or hospital. In the hospital setting, ambulatory procedures can be consolidated in one location or interspersed with inpatient procedures. Transportation between the procedural facility and a hospital for additional postoperative care also must be considered, and a transfer process should be in place. A facility that is accredited by the American Association for

Accreditation of Ambulatory Surgery Facilities, the Accreditation Association for Ambulatory Health Care, or the Joint Commission is essentially obliged to operate in a manner consistent with the American Society of Anesthesiologists (ASA) standards and guidelines. In addition to the physical plant, the available equipment and supplies will also influence what procedures may be performed. The ASA and others have set expectations for ambulatory anesthesia in the form of standards and guidelines that apply independent of location.[3] For example, the ASA and the Agency for Healthcare Research Quality recommend that equipment for standard monitoring include a noninvasive blood pressure monitor, a means to record heart rate and respiration, an electrocardiograph, and a pulse oximeter.[4] The ASA adds continuous monitoring of end expiratory carbon dioxide and the ability to measure temperature, if indicated.[5]

Safety is a continuum from the preoperative to the postoperative phase of care; at the time of discharge, patients should received written postoperative instructions and be discharged to the care of a responsible adult. Ideally, when surgery

Department of Anesthesia & Critical Care, The University of Chicago Medicine, 5841 S. Maryland Avenue, MC 4028, Chicago, IL 60637, USA
* Corresponding author.
E-mail address: jeffa@dacc.uchicago.edu

Clin Plastic Surg 40 (2013) 371–382
http://dx.doi.org/10.1016/j.cps.2013.04.004
0094-1298/13/$ – see front matter © 2013 Elsevier Inc. All rights reserved.

is performed in a freestanding ambulatory surgery center or office, the surgeon performing the surgery should have credentials to perform that procedure in a hospital and should be operating within the scope of his specialty training.

Another consideration is the personnel staffing the center. Will anesthesia be required, and if so, how much and administered by whom? Will a registered nurse be sufficient if anesthesia is given as a local injection with moderate sedation, or will the services of an anesthesiologist or a certified registered nurse anesthetist (CRNA) be needed? One study showed that anesthesia provided by nonanesthesiologists was associated with significantly higher rates of unexpected hospital admissions compared with that provided by solo anesthesiologists or a care team of physician and CRNA.[6] Who will perform the procedure? Will it be a physician, physician's assistant, or CRNA who may require physician supervision? Do the recovery room personnel have postanesthesia care experience commensurate with the type of anesthesia anticipated? Will they be able to handle possible complications from the procedure or the anesthetic? In summary, the staffing for all procedures should be adequate to meet the needs of the patient and the providers.[3]

Initially, ambulatory procedures were restricted to those associated with minimal blood loss that could be performed in less than 90 minutes with simple equipment, requiring minimal postoperative care and producing only mild pain that could be controlled with oral medications.[7] Now the only criterion strictly applied is that the patient is able to go home the same day of the procedure, although for some patients a 23-hour hospital stay or other nursing care environment is necessary.

The most complex variable is the patient, whose comorbidities determine whether a procedure may be performed in an ambulatory facility. In 1940, a classification scheme was created to standardize and define the operative risk of patients based on the history and physical examination.[8] Over the past 70 years, this original classification has been modified, with the current ASA physical status (PS) classification divided into 6 categories (**Box 1**). Although the ASA classification was not created originally as a predictive index of perioperative risk, it has been used as a proxy for risk in several studies.[9,10]

Overall surgical mortality for patients with ASA PS 1 through 3 is low (**Table 1**), but as PS class increases, so does the risk for morbidity. In a prospective analysis of 38,598 patients undergoing 45,090 ambulatory procedures, patients with ASA PS 3 constituted 24% of the morbidity.[11] In another study, an ASA PS rating of 2 or 3

Box 1
Classification of a patient's physical condition

1. A normal healthy patient.
2. A patient with mild systemic disease.
3. A patient with severe systemic disease.
4. A patient with severe systemic disease that is a constant threat to life.
5. A moribund patient who is not expected to survive without the operation.
6. A patient who has been declared brain-dead and whose organs are being removed for donor purposes.

---

predicted a 2-fold greater risk for unanticipated hospital admissions after ambulatory surgery.[12] A retrospective study of 28,921 patients undergoing ambulatory surgery found no significant difference in unplanned admissions between those with ASA PS 3 and those with ASA PS 1 and 2, although those with ASA PS 3 experienced more pain than patients with ASA PS 1 and 2.[13] Although patients with an ASA PS 1 through 3 have low risk with low rates (<2%) of postoperative complications,[12,13] the overall medical condition of a patient is the most important consideration,[14] and ASA PS alone should not determine eligibility for ambulatory surgery.

CARDIOVASCULAR DISEASE

The prevalence of coronary heart disease (CHD) in the United States is now 6%, with the greatest incidence in people 65 years of age or older (19.8%), followed by people aged 45 to 64 years (4.6%).[15] The overall mortality rates for patients with CHD have decreased since the 1960s, and this is attributable to improved medical

---

Table 1
American Society of Anesthesiologists classification and 30-day surgical mortality

ASA Physical Status Level	30-Day Mortality Rate (%)
1	0.0 ± 0.0
2	0.2 ± 0.1
3	2.2 ± 0.4
4	15.2 ± 2.4
5	70.0 ± 10.5

Data from Davenport DL, Bowe EA, Henderson WG, et al. National Surgical Quality Improvement Program (NSQIP) risk factors can be used to validate American Society of Anesthesiologists Physical Status Classification (ASA PS) Levels. Ann Surg 2006;243:636–44.

treatment.[16] In 2007, the American College of Cardiology (ACC) and the American Heart Association (AHA) published updated guidelines for cardiac evaluation and care for patients undergoing noncardiac surgery (**Fig. 1**).[17] For patients with unstable coronary syndromes, such as unstable or severe angina or recent myocardial infarction, decompensated heart failure, arrhythmias (high-grade or Mobitz II atrioventricular block, third-degree atrioventricular block, symptomatic ventricular arrhythmia, supraventricular arrhythmias with uncontrolled ventricular rate, symptomatic bradycardia, and newly recognized ventricular tachycardia), or severe valvular disease (severe aortic stenosis and symptomatic mitral stenosis), elective surgery should be delayed until further evaluation.[17] In a 1978 study of patients who had a myocardial infarction within 6 months before surgery, 27.3% experienced a perioperative infarction or cardiac death.[18] A 2012 study of the risk of perioperative myocardial infarction in 971,455 patients who had an infarction before surgery demonstrated that only 2% experienced a reinfarction.[19] Despite the apparent dramatic decrease in reinfarction, active cardiac symptoms do signal a risk.[20] For some patients, ambulatory surgery may not be a low-risk procedure.

A patient's functional status is the last criterion to be evaluated under the ACC/AHA algorithm. One metabolic equivalent (MET), the amount of oxygen consumed while sitting at rest, is equal to 3.5 mL of oxygen per kilogram of body weight per minute.[17] The threshold for good functional capacity is 4 METs (able to climb 1 flight of stairs or perform light housework). Patients who were not able to perform 4 METs during daily activities had increased perioperative and long-term risks, and an inverse relationship was seen between the number of blocks or flights a patient could walk and perioperative cardiovascular events.[21] If a patient does not have good functional capacity or is unable to perform 4 METs during daily activities, clinical predictors (eg, ischemic heart disease, heart failure, cerebrovascular disease, diabetes, renal insufficiency) and surgical risk will determine whether further perioperative testing is needed.[17]

For patients with cardiac stents, the ACC, AHA, and the American College of Surgeons have developed joint advisory recommendations for dual antiplatelet therapy. Patients with a bare metal stent should be treated with clopidogrel, 75 mg, and aspirin, 325 mg, for a minimum of 1 month, a sirolimus drug-eluting stent (DES) for a minimum of 3 months, and a paclitaxel DES for a minimum of 6 to 12 months to prevent stent thrombosis.[22] In a large observational study in which antiplatelet therapy was discontinued prematurely for patients with a DES, 29% of patients developed stent thrombosis.[23] Surgery is not recommended for at least 90 days after implantation of a bare metal stent. The odds ratio (OR) for a major cardiac event after surgery within 30 days of stent placement was 3.6, and was 1.6 for surgeries performed between 31 and 90 days of placement. For patients with DES implants, the rate of serious cardiac events was 5.7% to 6.6% for surgeries performed in fewer than 365 days from stent placement and 3.3% in surgeries after 365 days. A cardiologist should be consulted before discontinuation of antiplatelet therapy in these individuals. Patients who are on β-blocker therapy should continue these agents through the perioperative period.[17]

The ACC/AHA guidelines provide the tools to determine whether additional cardiac testing is required before surgery, and following the guidelines for antiplatelet and medical therapy further decreases patient risk. Individuals at high risk for perioperative cardiac events and those with recent myocardial infarctions or cardiac interventions may not be suitable for procedures in an ambulatory setting without access to interventional cardiology.

PULMONARY RISK FACTORS

Asthma affects 24.6 million people in the United States, or approximately 8.2% of the population.[24] Chronic obstructive pulmonary disease (COPD) is identified in at least 10 million adults, and the Centers for Disease Control and Prevention (CDC) believes it is underdiagnosed.[25] Although postoperative pulmonary complications are as prevalent as perioperative cardiac complications,[26] pulmonary risk stratification has only recently received attention.

Postoperative pulmonary complications increase length of hospital stay, morbidity, and mortality,[27] and in the case of ambulatory surgery, unplanned admissions. In one study of morbidity and mortality within 1 month of ambulatory surgery, respiratory failure constituted 16% of all morbidity.[11] In a respiratory risk index developed for respiratory failure after vascular or general surgery, respiratory failure was defined as postoperative mechanical ventilation for longer than 48 hours or unanticipated reintubation. Twenty-eight variables were independently associated with respiratory failure, including alcohol use (>2 drinks per day for 2 weeks before the procedure), greater than 10% weight loss in the previous 6 months, elevated blood urea nitrogen levels, low albumin levels, smoking, general anesthesia, and a surgical

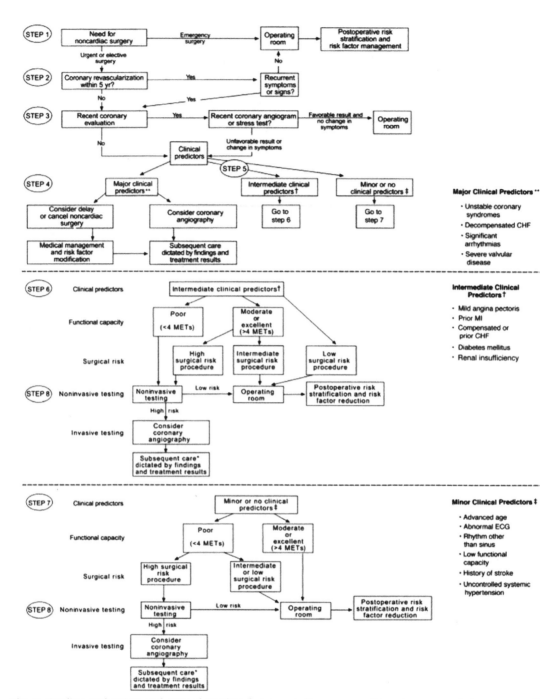

Fig. 1. Cardiac evaluation and care algorithm for noncardiac surgery. Stepwise approach to preoperative cardiac assessment. *Subsequent care may include cancellation or delay of surgery, coronary revascularization followed by noncardiac surgery, or intensified care. (*From* Eagle KA, Berger PB, Calkins H, et al. ACC/AHA guideline update for perioperative cardiovascular evaluation for noncardiac surgery—executive summary: a report of the American College of Cardiology/American Heart Association Task Force on Practice Guidelines (Committee to Update the 1996 Guidelines on Perioperative Cardiovascular Evaluation for Noncardiac Surgery). J Am Coll Cardiol 2002;39(3):542–53. http://dx.doi.org/10.1016/S0735-1097(01)01788-0; with permission.)

time from 2.5 to 4 hours.[27,28] The site and complexity of the operation are the most important factors for evaluating risk of respiratory failure. For procedures with relative value units (RVUs) from 10 to 17, such as orthopedic surgery, exploratory laparotomies, or hysterectomy, the OR for respiratory failure is 2.299 (confidence interval [CI], 1.937–2.728); for RVUs greater than 17 (eg, cardiac surgery, airway surgery, craniotomies), the OR is 4.445 (CI, 3.720–5.312). In other words, patients who undergo cardiac, thoracic, major vascular, or upper abdominal surgery, or head and neck procedures are at increased risk for postoperative respiratory failure.[29]

COPD is the most frequently identified risk factor for postoperative pulmonary complications,[26,30] such as atelectasis, pneumonia, respiratory failure, and exacerbation of underlying chronic lung disease. In an analysis of 15 studies, the OR was 1.79 (CI, 1.44–2.22) for pulmonary complications in patients with COPD.[26] Another study calculated an OR of 1.517 (CI, 1.362–1.689) for respiratory complications in patients with COPD,[27] and a Canadian study showed that COPD increased operative events by a factor of 2.[31] Patients are at highest risk in the immediate postoperative period from respiratory motor dysfunction, hypoxia, and hypoventilation,[32] and should be closely monitored. COPD in isolation is only a minor risk factor for postoperative respiratory failure.

Whether spirometry or chest radiographs help with pulmonary risk stratification or provide incrementally more information than the history and physical examination has not been determined,[26,28] and these tests should not be performed routinely for preoperative assessment. Guidelines from the American College of Physicians recommend that patients with stable COPD, irrespective of forced expiratory volume in the first second of expiration (FEV_1), be treated with inhaled bronchodilators. Patients with symptomatic COPD and an FEV_1 less than 60% of predicted percentage should be treated with either a long-acting inhaled anticholinergic or a long-acting inhaled β-agonist[33,34] and treatment should continue through the perioperative period. As for intraoperative management, a meta-analysis showed that spinal and epidural anesthetics decrease postoperative mortality, deep vein thrombosis, pneumonia, and respiratory depression.[35]

Even though the prevalence of asthma in the United States is increasing,[36,37] morbidity and mortality are decreasing because of advances in medical management.[37] Patients with asthma have varying degrees of airway obstruction, inflammation, and hyperresponsiveness. During anesthesia, aspiration, infection, instrumentation of the airway, the administration of certain drugs, or an inadequate depth of anesthesia may induce bronchospasm,[37] and patients with a history of asthma have a 5-fold risk of postoperative respiratory events.[38] Although perioperative bronchospasm is a concern, it occurs in only approximately 2% of patients.[37,38] As with patients with COPD, preoperative optimization is critical. Current guidelines indicate that inhaled corticosteroids are the most effective agents for long-term control of the disease.[39] Smoking cessation is a preoperative measure that can decrease the hyperreactivity of the airway, and not smoking for as few as 4 weeks preoperatively improves outcomes.[28] The American Thoracic Society and the European Respiratory Society recommend that patients cease smoking 6 to 8 weeks before surgery.[37]

Pulmonary risk factors alone do not predict postoperative pulmonary complications; the type of procedure and the surgical location are the most important predictors.[28,31] COPD is not an absolute contraindication to any surgery, but elective surgery should be postponed to treat an exacerbation of COPD or asthma. Well-controlled asthma does not increase risk for perioperative complications.[37,39]

ELDERLY PATIENTS

Currently in the United States, 39.6 million Americans are older than 65 years, and by 2030, the Census Bureau estimates the number will exceed 72.1 million.[40] Elderly patients may benefit greatly from an ambulatory procedure because they will be discharged home the day of surgery and may experience less cognitive impairment.[41] In addition to neurologic deterioration, aging causes physiologic changes in the body, including "vascular stiffening," which elevates blood pressure and increases pulse pressure. Unlike diastolic blood pressure (DBP), systolic blood pressure (SBP) increases an average of 6.2 mm Hg per decade,[42] and the prevalence of cardiovascular disease also increases with age.[43] In the lungs, elastic recoil diminishes, the chest wall stiffens, and motor power for respirations weakens in a smaller intervertebral space, all of which can promote atelectasis. Elderly people also have an impaired respiratory response to elevated carbon dioxide and hypoxia, making them more sensitive to the respiratory effects of narcotics and other anesthetic agents.[44,45]

Perioperative mortality increases with age, especially after emergency procedures or major surgery.[46] Elderly people are at greater risk for intraoperative events, such as hypertension, hypotension, and arrhythmia (OR, 1.42); intraoperative bleeding (OR, 1.31); and postoperative bruising (OR, 1.75),[47–49] but their risk for postoperative pain (OR, 0.2), shivering, nausea and vomiting (OR, 0.3), and desaturation (OR, 0.4) is less.[48] Patients older than 85 years with serious comorbidities are more likely to need hospital admission,[50] and elderly patients with a previous hospital admission within 6 months of the surgery have a 2-fold greater risk for unanticipated postoperative admission. Unanticipated hospital admissions rates after outpatient surgery remain at less than 3%.[41,50] Despite the risks, the overall mortality for elderly patients undergoing ambulatory procedures remains low. Of 564,267 outpatient surgical procedures in patients older than 65 years, the overall death rate per 100,000 was 2.3 on the day of the procedure, 5.1 on days 1 to 7 afterward, and 6.6 on days 8 to 30.[50]

Despite physiologic changes in the elderly, ambulatory surgery has proven to be safe, which can be attributed to careful patient selection via a thorough preoperative assessment.[45] To evaluate an elderly patient for ambulatory surgery, consideration is given to the type of surgery, the surgical and anesthetic risk, and the functional capacity of the patient. The medical condition of the patient is optimized before surgery to minimize risk and reduce the likelihood of adverse events.[51–53] As with all patients, the social situation should be evaluated to determine whether the elderly patient has help at home for postoperative care.[41]

Hypertension

In the United States, 1 in 3 individuals has hypertension. Although men younger than 45 years have a higher prevalence, the percentages of men and women equalize thereafter.[54] In people older than 65 years, the prevalence increases to more than 50%.[55] The diagnosis of hypertension requires, "the average of two or more properly measured, seated blood pressure readings on each of two or more office visits."[56] Stage 1 hypertension is a SBP of 140 to 159 mm Hg or a DBP of 90 to 99 mm Hg. Stage 2 is an SBP greater than or equal to 160 mm Hg or DBP greater than or equal to 100 mm Hg.[56] Although not described in the updated National Institutes of Health model of 2007, the literature describes stage 3 of hypertension as an SBP greater than or equal to 180 mm Hg or DBP greater than or equal to 110 mm Hg.[17]

Hypertension in outpatient surgery has not been extensively studied, and most of the outcome data have come from the studies conducted on inpatients. Beyer and colleagues[57] evaluated 125,000 procedures over 5 years and found that patients with hypertension had a 40% increased risk of

an intraoperative arrhythmia or hemodynamic abnormalities. Wax and colleagues[58] found that increased levels of preinduction SBP and DBP were an independent risk factor for postoperative myocardial injury, infarction, or death. In the outpatient setting, Chung and colleagues[48] found that hypertension was associated with increased intraoperative events, primarily cardiovascular, and included hypertension, arrhythmias, hypotension, tachycardia, and bradycardia. It was also associated with increased postoperative events, including hematoma. They recommend careful preoperative blood pressure control and perioperative management. This recommendation is consistent with the 2007 ACC/AHA guidelines that state if a patient presents for initial evaluation with stage 1 or 2 hypertension and has no end-organ disease or associated metabolic abnormalities, there is no reason to delay surgery. The meta-analysis by Howell and colleagues[59] further supports the ACC/AHA recommendation, which found insufficient evidence of an association between SBP less than 180 mm Hg and DBP less than 100 mm Hg and perioperative complications. However, the ACC/AHA guidelines recommend that elective surgery be postponed for patients with stage 3 hypertension to improve blood pressure control over several days or even weeks.[17] Although the literature does not have any consensus about delaying or canceling surgery for stage 3 hypertension, it does suggest that hypertension should not be looked at in isolation when determining whether to proceed, and that it need not be regarded as an absolute contraindication. For patients with end-organ damage induced by hypertension (eg, ischemic heart disease, heart failure, renal or cerebrovascular disease) whose perioperative risk would be substantially decreased by delaying the procedure, hypertension management should be considered. In addition, the urgency or necessity of the procedure should be taken into consideration.[60]

OBSTRUCTIVE SLEEP APNEA

Approximately 2% to 25% of the general population has obstructive sleep apnea (OSA)[61] and may have other comorbidities, such as hypertension and obesity.[62] Because of a concern for possible perioperative complications, a question exists about the appropriateness of allowing patients with OSA to undergo ambulatory surgery.

Individuals with OSA have physical alterations of the lateral pharyngeal walls and tongue. Their computed tomography and magnetic resonance imaging studies reveal fat deposits and submucosal edema, which narrow the pharyngeal airway.[63] During awake respiration, activity of the upper airway dilator muscle counteracts the effect of a narrowed airway,[63] but inhaled anesthetics and narcotics collapse the airway. Narcotics can exacerbate the problem through inducing central apnea.[64]

OSA is an independent risk factor for morbidity and mortality.[65] Among postoperative complications of patients with OSA, oxygen desaturation is the most common[62] and more likely to occur immediately after extubation than later in the postanesthesia care unit.[66] Postoperative hypoxia does not seem to result in increased mortality, unanticipated hospital admission, or delay in discharge.[65,67,68] A meta-analysis by the Society of Ambulatory Anesthesia (SAMBA) found no increase in mortality and no correlation between adverse events and clinically significant adverse outcomes. Despite postoperative hypoxemia, no intubation or ventilator assistance was required.[67]

In a consensus statement on preoperative selection of patients with OSA scheduled for ambulatory surgery, SAMBA recommended screening patients with the STOP BANG questionnaire because it is simple to administer (**Box 2**) and accurately predicts the probability that a patient has moderate to severe OSA. A STOP BANG score of 5 had an OR of 4.5 for moderate/severe OSA and an OR of 10.4 for severe OSA. A score of 7 to 8 had an OR of 6.9 for moderate/severe OSA and an OR of 14.9 for severe OSA.[69] **Fig. 2** presents a decision-making algorithm for preoperative selection.

Box 2
The STOP BANG questionnaire

S = Snoring: do you snore loudly (louder than talking or loud enough to be heard through closed doors)?

T = Tiredness: do you often feel tired fatigued, or sleepy during daytime?

O = Observed apnea: has anyone ever observed you stop breathing during your sleep?

P = Pressure: do you have or are you being treated for high blood pressure?

B = BMI >35 kg/m^2

A = Age >50 years

N = Neck circumference >40 cm

G = Gender male

Low risk for OSA: <3 questions positive.

High risk of OSA: ≥3 questions positive.

High probability of moderate to severe OSA: 5–8 questions positive.

DIABETES MELLITUS

In the United States, 8.3% of the population has been diagnosed with diabetes, with approximately 1.9 million new diagnoses every year.[70] Because people with diabetes require more surgical procedures than those without,[71] they are often cared for in an ambulatory surgery center. Many of the recommendations for glucose management in patients with diabetes undergoing ambulatory surgery have been extrapolated from studies of inpatient surgeries.[72]

A hyperglycemic condition can cause metabolic derangements, including dehydration, electrolyte abnormalities, and ketoacidosis.[73] The stress response of surgery triggers the release of epinephrine, norepinephrine, cortisol, glucagon, and growth hormones.[71,74] These catabolic hormones combine with the inhibited insulin secretion that results from the stress response to raise blood glucose levels in the perioperative period.[71,74] As with inpatients, the main objective in management is to preserve glucose control and prevent hypoglycemia.[74] Pharmacologic treatment of patients with diabetes includes oral hypoglycemic medications, long- or short-acting insulin, or a combination of the aforementioned agents. Patients taking oral hypoglycemic medications should be instructed to take their medications as they normally would on the day before surgery, but these agents should be discontinued on the day of surgery. Patients taking long-acting or intermediate-acting insulin take their prescribed doses while eating a normal diet.[75] On the day of surgery, patients who take intermediate-acting agents (eg, neutral protamine Hagedorn insulin [NPH], Lente) may need to decrease or discontinue the dose, because they may experience hypoglycemia if a meal is omitted.[72] Patients taking long-acting insulin agents reduce the dose on the day of surgery.

On the day of surgery, blood glucose should minimally be measured on the patient's arrival at the surgical facility and postoperatively. If the surgical procedure is prolonged, blood glucose levels should be checked intraoperatively.[71] Consensus has not been reached on an optimal intraoperative blood glucose level, but the NICE-SUGAR study found that patients with a blood glucose level less than 180 mg/dL had a lower mortality rate than those whose glucose level was tightly controlled between 81 and 108 mg/dL.[76]

Diabetes in and of itself is not a contraindication to ambulatory surgery, but patients with diabetes often have other comorbidities, such as hypertension, dyslipidemia, obesity, and chronic kidney disease. The evaluation of a patient's medical status determines whether an ambulatory setting is

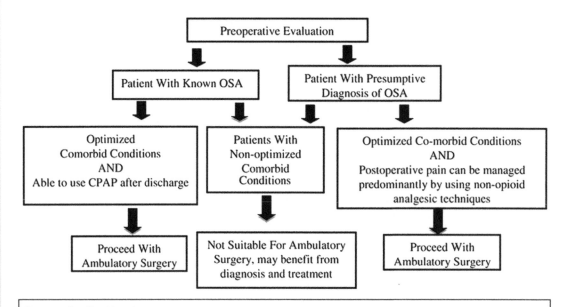

Fig. 2. Decision-making algorithm for patients with OSA.

OBESITY

Obesity is defined as a body mass index (BMI) greater than 30 kg/m^2; morbid obesity is a BMI greater than 40 kg/m^2.[77] The CDC reports that by the year 2030, 42% of Americans will be obese. The CDC also predicts that in 2030 the severely obese will constitute 11% of the population.[78] Obese patients are likely to have hypertension, coronary artery disease, OSA, asthma, diabetes, and metabolic syndrome. Obesity alone is not a risk factor for unanticipated admissions after ambulatory surgery,[79] but obese patients have a statistically significant higher incidence of intraoperative bronchospasm than nonobese patients

appropriate for the procedure. If a surgical facility is going to care for patients with diabetes, it must have the necessary equipment to test and monitor blood glucose levels.

and require supplemental oxygen postoperatively.[79] The patient's comorbidities, the anesthetic required, and the type of surgery determine whether a patient is a candidate for a procedure in an ambulatory setting.

PREOPERATIVE TESTING

Screening laboratory tests have not been shown to be useful and are likely a waste of resources. Preoperative tests for screening purposes tend to be nonspecific and do not change the anesthetic management of the patient in the ambulatory setting.[80] Studies have has also demonstrated that eliminating routine testing does not increase risk.[81] A study of 1061 patients randomized to undergo either directed preoperative testing or no preoperative testing showed no significant difference in rates of adverse events between ambulatory surgical groups. The authors concluded that testing may be safely eliminated in selected patients.[82,83]

SUMMARY

Ambulatory surgery is commonplace for a multitude of procedures and a wide range of patients. The types of procedures performed in the ambulatory setting are becoming more work-intensive, and patients with comorbidities make for a challenging environment. For a safe environment for surgery in ambulatory facilities, the complex task of patient selection is necessary. Until an algorithm is created that includes provider, procedure, facility, and patient comorbidites, clinicians must rely on general guidelines rather than precise recommendations. When determining whether a patient is suitable for ambulatory surgery, multiple factors must be assessed. The surgical procedure, who will be performing the surgical procedures, whether anesthesia is required, the type of anesthesia provider (eg, conscious sedation with a surgeon and nurse, an anesthesiologist, or a CRNA), and the surgical setting (eg, hospital-based ambulatory surgical center vs free-standing surgical center vs a physician's office) all must be taken into account. In addition to these factors, patients and their comorbidities must be considered. Individual medical problems (eg, coronary artery disease, COPD, diabetes) taken in isolation often are not absolute contraindications to ambulatory surgery; patients must be evaluated as a whole to determine whether the procedure can be performed on an ambulatory basis.

REFERENCES

1. MEDPAC Report to the Congress: Medicare Payment Policy. 2004.
2. Cullen KA, Hall MJ, Golosinskiy A. Ambulatory surgery in the United States, 2006. Natl Health Stat Report 2009;11:1–28.
3. Guidelines for ambulatory anesthesia and surgery. American Society of Anesthesiologists Web site. Available at: http://www.asahq.org/For-Healthcare-Professionals/Standards-Guidelines-and-Statements.aspx. Accessed August 31, 2012.
4. Evidence-based patient safety advisory: patient selection and procedures in ambulatory surgery. Agency for Healthcare Research and Quality Web site. Available at: http://guidelines.gov/content.aspx?id=15334. Accessed September 1, 2012.
5. Standards for basic anesthetic monitoring. American Society of Anesthesiologists Web site. Available at: http://www.asahq.org/For-Healthcare-Professionals/Standards-Guidelines-and-Statements.aspx. Accessed September 10, 2012.
6. Memtsoudis SG, Ma Y, Swamidoss CP, et al. Factors influencing unexpected disposition after orthopedic ambulatory surgery. J Clin Anesth 2012;24:89–95.
7. White PF. Outpatient anesthesia. New York: Churchill Livingstone; 1990. p. 2–5.
8. Schwam SJ, Gold MI, Craythorne NW. The ASA physical status classification: a revision. Anesthesiology 1962;577:A439.
9. Voney G, Biro P, Roos M, et al. Interrelation of perioperative morbidity and ASA class assignment in patients undergoing gynaecological surgery. Eur J Obstet Gynecol Reprod Biol 2007;132:220–5.
10. Davenport DL, Bowe EA, Henderson WG, et al. National Surgical Quality Improvement Program (NSQIP) risk factors can be used to validate American Society of Anesthesiologists Physical Status Classification (ASA PS) levels. Ann Surg 2006;243:636–44.
11. Warner MA, Shields SE, Chute CG. Major morbidity and mortality within 1 month of ambulatory surgery and anesthesia. JAMA 1993;270:1437–41.
12. Fortier J, Chung F, Su J. Unanticipated admission after ambulatory surgery—a prospective study. Can J Anaesth 1998;45:612–9.
13. Ansell GL, Montgomery JE. Outcome of ASA III patients undergoing day case surgery. Br J Anaesth 2004;92:71–4.
14. Verma R, Alladi R, Jackson I, et al. Guidelines: day case and short stay surgery: 2. Anaesthesia 2011;66:417–34.
15. Centers for Disease Control and Prevention (CDC). Prevalence of coronary heart disease—United States 2006-2010. MMWR Morb Mortal Wkly Rep 2011;60:1377–81.
16. Xu JQ, Kochanek KD, Murphy SL, et al. Deaths: final data for 2007. Natl Vital Stat Rep 2010;58(19):1–135.
17. Fleisher LA, Beckman JA, Brown KA, et al. ACC/AHA 2007 guidelines on perioperative cardiovascular evaluation and care for noncardiac surgery: a report of the American College of Cardiology/American Heart Association Task Force on Practice Guidelines (Writing Committee to Revise the 2002 Guidelines on Perioperative Cardiovascular Evaluation for Noncardiac Surgery). J Am Coll Cardiol 2007;50:e159–241.
18. Goldman L, Claldera DL, Soutwick FS, et al. Cardiac risk factors and complications in non-cardiac surgery. Medicine 1978;57:357–70.
19. Larsen KD, Rubinfeld IS. Changing risk of perioperative myocardial infarction. Perm J 2012;16:4–9.
20. Sweitzer BJ. Preoperative screening, evaluation, and optimization of the patient's medical status before outpatient surgery. Curr Opin Anaesthesiol 2008;21:711–8.

21. Reilly DF, McNeely MJ, Doerner D, et al. Self –reported exercise tolerance and the risk of serious perioperative complications. Arch Intern Med 1999;159:2185–92.

22. Grines CL, Bonow RO, Case DE, et al. Antiplatelet therapy in patients with coronary artery stents. A science advisory from the American Heart Association, the American College of Cardiology, Society for Cardiovascular Angiography and Interventions, American College of Surgeons, and American Dental Association, with representation from the American College of Physicians. J Am Coll Cardiol 2007;49:734–9.

23. Iakovou I, Schmidt T, Bonizzoni E, et al. Incidence, predictors and outcome of thrombosis after successful implantation of drug-eluting stents. JAMA 2005;293:2126–30.

24. Akinbami L, Moorman JE, Liu X. Asthma prevalence, health care use, and mortality: United States, 2005-2009. Natl Health Stat Report 2011;(32): 1–14.

25. Mannino DM, Homa DM, Akinbami LJ, et al. Chronic obstructive pulmonary disease surveillance–United States, 1971-2000. MMWR Surveill Summ 2001;51: 1–16.

26. Smetana G, Lawrence VA, Cornell JE. Preoperative pulmonary risk stratification for noncardiothoracic surgery: systematic review for the American College of Physicians. Ann Intern Med 2006;144: 581–95.

27. Johnson RG, Arozullah AM, Neumayer L, et al. Multivariable predictors of postoperative respiratory failure after general and vascular surgery: results from the Patient Safety in Surgery Study. J Am Coll Surg 2007;204:1188–98.

28. Smetana GW, Conde M. Preoperative pulmonary update. Clin Geriatr Med 2008;24:607–24.

29. Arozullah AM, Khuri SF, Henderson WG, et al. Development and validation of a multifactorial risk index for predicting postoperative pneumonia after major noncardiac surgery. Ann Intern Med 2001; 135:846–57.

30. Smetana GW. Preoperative pulmonary evaluation. N Engl J Med 1999;340:937–44.

31. Wong DH, Weber EC, Schell MJ, et al. Factors associated with postoperative pulmonary complications in patients with severe chronic obstructive pulmonary disease. Anesth Analg 1995;80: 276–84.

32. Duncan PG, Cohen MM, Tweed WA, et al. The Canadian four-centre study of anaesthetic outcomes: III. Are anaesthetic complications predictable in day surgical practice? Can J Anaesth 1992; 39(5 Pt 1):440–8.

33. Qaseem A, Wilt TJ, Weinberger SE, et al. Diagnosis and management of stable chronic obstructive pulmonary disease: a clinical practice guideline update from the American College of Physicians, American College of Chest Physicians, American Thoracic Society, and European Respiratory Society. Ann Intern Med 2011;155:181–91.

34. Standards of the diagnosis and management of patients with COPD. American Thoracic Society Web site. Available at: http://www.thoracic.org/clinical/copd-guidelines/index.php. Accessed September 8, 2012.

35. Rodgers A, Walker N, Schug S, et al. Reduction of postoperative mortality and morbidity with epidural or spinal anesthesia: results from overview of randomized trials. BMJ 2000;321:1493–7.

36. Chung F, Mezei G. Factors contributing to a prolonged stay after ambulatory surgery. Anesth Analg 1999;89:1352–9.

37. Centers for Disease Control and Prevention (CDC). Vital signs: asthma prevalence, disease characteristics, and self-management education—United States, 2001-2009. MMWR Morb Mortal Wkly Rep 2011;60:547–52.

38. Woods BD, Sladen RN. Perioperative considerations for the patient with asthma and bronchospasm. Br J Anaesth 2009;103:i57–65.

39. National Institutes of Health, National Heart Lung and Blood Institute. Expert panel report 3: guidelines for the diagnosis and management of asthma. Bethesda (MD): US Department of Health and Human Services. National Institutes of Health, National Heart, Lung, and Blood Institute; 2007. Available at: http://www.nhlbi.nih.gov/guidelines/asthma/asthgdln.pdf. Accessed September 9, 2012.

40. Older Americans 2012: Key Indicators of Well Being. Federal Interagency Forum on Aging Related Statistics. Available at: http://www.agingstats.gov/agingstatsdotnet/main_site/default.aspx. Accessed August 12, 2012.

41. Mattila K, Vironen J, Eklund A, et al. Randomized clinical trial comparing ambulatory and inpatient care after inguinal hernia repair in patients aged 65 years or older. Am J Surg 2011;201: 179–85.

42. Chen CH, Nakayama M, Nevo E, et al. Coupled systolic-ventricular and vascular stiffening with age implications for pressure regulation and cardiac reserve in the elderly. J Am Coll Cardiol 1998;32:1221–7.

43. Betelli G. Anaesthesia for the elderly outpatient: preoperative assessment and evaluation, anesthetic technique and postoperative pain management. Curr Opin Anaesthesiol 2010;23:726–31.

44. Wahba WM. Influence of aging on lung function—clinical significance of changes from age twenty. Anesth Analg 1983;62:764–76.

45. White PF, White LM, Monk T, et al. Perioperative care for the older outpatient undergoing ambulatory surgery. Anesth Analg 2012;114:1190–215.

46. Jin F, Chung F. Minimizing perioperative adverse events in the elderly. Br J Anaesth 2001;87:608–24.

47. Chung F, Mezei G, Tong D. Adverse events in ambulatory survey. A comparison between elderly and younger patients. Can J Anaesth 1999;46:309–21.

48. Chung F, Mezei G, Tong D. Pre-existing medical conditions as predictors of adverse events in day case surgery. Br J Anaesth 1999;83:262–70.

49. Cutter PL, Trinhaus KM. Hemorrhagic complications of oculoplastic surgery. Ophthal Plast Reconstr Surg 2002;18:409–15.

50. Fleisher LA, Pasternak LR, Herbert R, et al. Inpatient hospital admission and death after outpatient surgery in elderly patients. Importance of patient and system characteristics and location of care. Arch Surg 2004;139:67–72.

51. Shnaider I, Chung F. Outcomes in day surgery. Curr Opin Anaesthesiol 2006;19:622–9.

52. McGory ML, Kao KK, Shekelle PG, et al. Developing quality indicators for elderly surgical patients. Ann Surg 2009;260:338–47.

53. Jakobsson J. Ambulatory anaesthesia: there is room for further improvements of safety and quality of care—is the way forward further simply one of evidence-based risk scores? Curr Opin Anaesthesiol 2010;23:670–81.

54. Holmes JS, Kozak LJ, Owings MF. Use and in-hospital mortality associated with two cardiac procedures, by sex and age: National Trends, 1990-2003. Health Aff 2007;26:169–77.

55. Roger VL, Go AS, Lloyd-Jones DM, et al. Heart disease and stroke statistics—2012 update. A report from the American Heart Association. Circulation 2012;125:e2–220.

56. Seventh Report of the Joint National Committee on Prevention, Detection, Evaluation, and Treatment of High Blood Pressure (JNC 7 Express). Available at: http://www.nhlbi.nih.gov/guidelines/hypertension/jnc7full.pdf. Accessed November 25, 2012.

57. Beyer K, Taffe P, Halfon P, et al. Hypertension and intra-operative incidents: a multicenter study of 125000 surgical procedures in Swiss Hospitals. Anaesthesia 2009;64:494–502.

58. Wax DB, Porter SB, Lin HM, et al. Association of preanesthesia hypertension with adverse outcomes. J Cardiothorac Vasc Anesth 2010;24:927–30.

59. Howell SJ, Sear JW, Foex P. Hypertension, hypertensive heart disease and perioperative cardiac Risk. Br J Anaesth 2004;92:570–83.

60. Hanada S, Kawakami H, Goto T, et al. Hypertension and anesthesia. Curr Opin Anaesthesiol 2006;19:315–9.

61. Young T, Hutton R, Finn L, et al. The gender bias in sleep apnea diagnosis. Are women missed because they have different symptoms? Arch Intern Med 1996;156:2445–51.

62. Liao P, Yegneswaran B, Vairavanthan S, et al. Postoperative complications in patients with obstructive sleep apnea: a retrospective matched cohort study. Can J Anaesth 2009;56:819–28.

63. Patil SP, Schneider H, Schwartz AR. Adult obstructive sleep apnea pathophysiology and diagnosis. Chest 2007;132:325–37.

64. Waters KA, McBrien F, Stewart P, et al. Effects of OSA, inhalational anesthesia and fentanyl on the airway and ventilation of children. J Appl Physiol 2002;92:1986–94.

65. Sabers C, Plevak DJ, Schroeder DR, et al. The diagnosis of obstructive sleep apnea as a risk factor for unanticipated admissions in outpatient surgery. Anesth Analg 2003;96:1328–35.

66. Liu SS, Chisholm MF, John RS, et al. Risk of postoperative hypoxemia in ambulatory orthopedic surgery patients with diagnosis of obstructive sleep apnea: a retrospective observational study. Patient Saf Surg 2010;4:9–13.

67. Joshi GP, Ankichetty SP, Gan TJ, et al. Society for Ambulatory Anesthesia consensus statement on preoperative selection of adult patients with obstructive sleep apnea scheduled for ambulatory surgery. Anesth Analg 2012;115(5):1060–8.

68. Kurrek MM, Cobourn C, Wojtasik Z, et al. Morbidity in patients with or high risk for obstructive sleep apnea after ambulatory laparoscopic gastric banding. Obes Surg 2011;21:1494–8.

69. Chung F, Subramanyam R, Liao P, et al. High STOP-Bang score indicates a high probability of obstructive sleep apnoea. Br J Anaesth 2012;108:768–75.

70. Diabetes statistics. American Diabetes Association Web site. Available at: http://www.diabetes.org/diabetes-basics/diabetes-statistics/. Accessed October 5, 2012.

71. Dagogo-Jack S, Alberti K. Management of diabetes mellitus in surgical patients. Diabetes Spectr 2002;15:44–8.

72. Joshi GP, Chung F, Vann MA, et al. Society for Ambulatory Anesthesia consensus statement on perioperative blood glucose management in diabetic patients undergoing ambulatory surgery. Anesth Analg 2010;111:1378–87.

73. Akhtar S, Barash PG, Inzucchi SE. Scientific principles and clinical implications of perioperative glucose regulation and control. Anesth Analg 2010;110:478–97.

74. Sheehy AM, Gabbay RA. An overview of preoperative glucose evaluation, management and perioperative impact. J Diabetes Sci Technol 2009;3:1262–9.

75. Vann MA. Perioperative management of ambulatory surgical patients with diabetes mellitus. Curr Opin Anaesthesiol 2009;22:718–24.

76. The NICE-SUGAR Study Investigators. Intensive versus conventional glucose control in critically ill patients. N Engl J Med 2009;360:1283–97.

77. Cullen A, Ferguson A. Perioperative management of the severely obese patient: a selective pathophysiological review. Can J Anaesth 2012;59(10): 974–96.

78. Ogden CL, Carroll MD, Kit BK, et al. Prevalence of obesity in the United States, 2009-2010. NCHS Data Brief 2012;82:1–8.

79. Hofer RE, Kai T, Decker P, et al. Obesity as a risk factor for unanticipated admissions after ambulatory surgery. Mayo Clin Proc 2008;83:908–13.

80. Richman DC. Ambulatory surgery: how much testing do we need? Anesthesiol Clin 2010;28:185–97.

81. Schein OD, Katz J, Bass EB, et al. The value of routine preoperative medical testing before cataract surgery. Study of Medical Testing for Cataract Surgery. N Engl J Med 2000;342(3):168–75.

82. Chung F, Yuan H, Yin L, et al. Elimination of preoperative testing in ambulatory surgery. Anesth Analg 2009;108:467–75.

83. Fleisher LA, Bechman AJ, Brown KA, et al. ACC/AHA 2007 guidelines on perioperative cardiovascular evaluation and care for noncardiac surgery. Circulation 2007;116:e418–500.

Conscious Sedation/Local Anesthesia in the Office-Based Surgical and Procedural Facility

Harlan Pollock, MD[a,b,c],*, Susan Forman, CRNA[a],
Todd Pollock, MD[a,b,c], Mark Raccasi, MD[a,c]

KEYWORDS

- Balanced anesthesia • Conscious sedation • Propofol • Constant infusion • Titration infusion
- Twilight sleep

KEY POINTS

- Conscious sedation/local anesthesia is a challenging technique requiring cooperation of the patient, surgeon, and anesthesia provider.
- The anesthesia provider keeps the patient sedated, whereas the surgeon provides the anesthesia (local).
- In the authors' experience, the defining factor of "conscious sedation" is the ability of the patient to maintain spontaneous respirations and the ability (reflexes) to protect the airway throughout the procedure.
- The properties of propofol, especially the rapid onset and short duration of action, make it an ideal agent for conscious sedation.
- Because the level of sedation can deepen unexpectedly with propofol, an anesthesia provider should administer and monitor the patient.
- Low-dose propofol conscious sedation with local anesthesia is a safe and effective anesthetic for a wide spectrum of surgical procedures.
- It is the dose of the drug, not the route of administration, which determines depth of sedation.
- PONV is infrequent with this technique.

With the increasing number of office-based surgical (OBS), medical, and diagnostic procedures done each year, there has been resurgence in the use of intravenous sedation. The American Association for the Accreditation of Ambulatory Surgical Facilities (AAAASF), which provides accreditation for most OBS and office-based medical facilities in the United States, has demonstrated the safety of OBS from peer review data involving more than 1 million procedures.[1] Several independent reports have confirmed the safety of ambulatory surgery.[2–5]

Current anesthetic methods, improved monitoring technology, and newer drugs have improved the safety of general anesthesia and that of intravenous sedation. The importance of OBS facility accreditation and appropriate physician credentialing for patient safety cannot be overemphasized and are integral to the conclusions of this article. In fact, when propofol is used, AAAASF requires a

Funding Sources: None.
Conflict of Interest: None.
[a] Texas Institute for Surgery, 7115 Greenville Avenue, Suite 100, Dallas, TX 75231, USA; [b] Department of Plastic Surgery, U.T. Southwestern Medical School, 5323 Harry Hines Boulevard, Dallas, TX 75235, USA; [c] T.H.R. Presbyterian Hospital of Dallas, 8300 Walnut Hill Lane, Dallas, Texas 75231, USA
* Corresponding author. 8305 Walnut Hill Lane, Suite 210, Dallas, TX 75231, USA.
E-mail address: hp@drpollock.com

Clin Plastic Surg 40 (2013) 383–388
http://dx.doi.org/10.1016/j.cps.2013.04.014
0094-1298/13/$ – see front matter © 2013 Elsevier Inc. All rights reserved.

credentialed anesthesia provider to administer the anesthetic and that the facility be equipped comparably with one approved for general anesthesia.

Intravenous sedation encompasses a broad continuum of levels of consciousness, from a low-dose tranquilizer reducing anxiety in an awake patient, to deep sedation requiring supplemental oxygen and airway management. Measurable outcomes of conscious sedation (midazolam/fentanyl) and deep (propofol) sedation have been found to be effective and safe in a series reported by Hansen and coworkers.[6] This article presents the authors' extensive experience with conscious sedation/local anesthesia as a safe, comfortable, and effective but constantly evolving technique. Because conscious sedation requires teamwork, the discussion includes the perspective of the various members of the operating room (OR) team.

CONSCIOUS SEDATION DEFINED

According to the American Society of Anesthesia, "Conscious sedation is a drug-induced depression of consciousness during which patients respond purposefully to verbal commands, either alone or accompanied by light tactile stimulation. No interventions are required to maintain a patent airway, and spontaneous ventilation is adequate. Cardiovascular function is usually maintained."[7] This is in contrast to deep sedation, in which the patient is unconscious and requires assistance with airway management, with potential impairment of cardiovascular function. Many surgeons prefer deep sedation because it requires less time and concern for patient comfort than conscious sedation. However, deep sedation increases the risk of airway compromise, incidence of postoperative nausea and vomiting (PONV), and recovery time. It could be argued that deep sedation is merely a "light general anesthetic" and should be treated as such with mechanical control of the airway. Conscious sedation, properly administered, is safer, has a lower incidence of PONV, and provides a shorter recovery.

In the authors' experience, the defining factor of conscious sedation is the ability of the patient to maintain spontaneous respirations and the ability (reflex) to protect the airway. Although the authors' patients are generally responsive to verbal and physical stimuli most of the time, they are maintained at a deeper level during the initial injection of the local anesthesia and occasionally and briefly at intervals of more intense stimulation. Occasionally, it is necessary to lift the jaw to temporarily maintain the airway, but the need to use a mask for positive pressure assistance was uncommon in the authors' series. In their experience, supplemental oxygen, which is potentially dangerous because of fire hazard, is not required, because no patient has exhibited hypoxia requiring the use of intubation.[8] Intraoral and intranasal airways are not routinely used. Of interest, Stemp has suggested that supplemental oxygen can actually be detrimental because it can mask and delay the diagnosis of hypoventilation.[9]

Conscious sedation/local anesthesia is a challenging technique requiring cooperation between the surgeon and anesthesia provider. The non-threatening office environment, with limited anesthesia equipment, recovery space, and personnel requirements, together with the reduced incidence of PONV and shorter recovery time, make this technique ideal for OSB procedures. Significantly, certain risks of general anesthesia can be reduced or avoided with the use of conscious sedation, including deep vein thrombosis, pulmonary complications, OR fires, and pressure injuries. The cost effectiveness of OBS and conscious sedation is crucial as hospital costs increase, despite shrinking health care resources. In cosmetic surgery, the use of conscious sedation and OBS can provide a valuable marketing advantage to the surgeon, including safety, cost, and patient satisfaction.[10] Empirically, the risk of deep venous thrombosis in a sedated patient should be negligible compared with general anesthesia. However, it is the authors' practice and an AAAASF requirement to use a sequential compression device on all cases lasting longer than an hour.

In some practices, oral sedation is used for OBS to avoid the necessity of accreditation, which is mandated in many states for facilities using intravenous sedation. However, most oral drugs have relatively long onset and duration, making the control of level of consciousness unpredictable. Furthermore, the occurrence of an overdose is difficult to manage without trained personnel and the availability of adequate resuscitation drugs and equipment. AAAASF requires the continual monitoring of vital signs, oxygenation, and continuous monitoring of electrocardiogram by a qualified physician when using sedation. It is important to understand that the depth of sedation is related to dose, not route of administration of the sedating drug.

CLINICAL EXPERIENCE

Fifteen years experience of 1400 consecutive cases done by a nurse anesthetist in a single practice Class B AAAASF OBS facility were retrospectively reviewed for incidence of anesthetic complications, fatalities, and unanticipated hospital admissions. Drugs used, doses given, and order of administration varied; however, the technique described here has evolved over the past 15 years and has proved effective and safe. **Table 1** shows the low incidence of complications of conscious sedation with local anesthesia. Several series have been published that mirror these data and conclusions.[1,3,4,10,11] Our data show that the routine use of supplemental oxygen for patients under conscious sedation is unnecessary. However, if the anesthesia provider prefers the use of supplemental oxygen, recent studies suggest a nasopharyngeal catheter may be safer than other delivery methods.[12]

No oral premedication was used in this technique because the authors and others have found oral medication can prolong recovery time and PONV. The authors' current conscious sedation technique uses low-dose propofol titration in combination with several other drugs, with effective sedation and short recovery period. Yoon and coworkers[11] describe propofol as the ideal sedative drug for local anesthesia in the ambulatory setting because it provides sedation, anxiolysis, and amnesia with rapid onset and recovery and few side effects. With low-dose propofol, careful titration and continual observation are necessary to achieve the desired level of consciousness, maintenance of airway, and respiratory drive. A constant infusion pump can be used with the benefit of more even levels of altered consciousness, but often results in deeper sedation.[4,13,14] Because of the potential for a rapid and unexpected deepening of sedation, only an anesthesia professional should administer propofol. It is important to advise patients that they may have some vague memories after conscious sedation,

rarely unpleasant, and usually from late in the procedure.

CONSCIOUS SEDATION TECHNIQUE

The technique described has been successfully used balancing doses of propofol, midazolam, fentanyl, and other adjuvants to achieve a safe level of sedation. The success of this technique has been a product of the continuous communication and cooperation between the surgeon, patient, and anesthesia provider. On the continuum of conscious to deep sedation, the technique described keeps the patient predominately in a conscious state with deeper sedation only at appropriate times and for short intervals.

The patient is contacted the day before surgery to discuss the proposed anesthetic management, to allay any concerns, and to explain the sedation experience. Referring to the anesthetic technique as "twilight sleep" is a term best understood by patients. The morning of surgery is an opportune time for the anesthesia provider to reassure the patient that they will not feel pain or experience anxiety during the procedure and likely will have no memory of the procedure. An explanation of a forthcoming maneuver, especially if it is uncomfortable, is key to avoiding surprises that might undermine any previously established confidence. Patient comfort, in and of itself, is reassuring, so appropriate room temperature, positioning, and assistance in transfer to the OR table should be a part of the preoperative management (**Fig. 1**).

After an intravenous line is established, medications are administered with an initial dose of midazolam, 0.025 mg/kg, and droperidol, 0.625 mg. This is followed by an initial dose of propofol, 0.5 mg/kg, and titration is continued until the patient no longer responds to verbal stimuli. Close observation of the patient response is key in

Table 1 Complications	
Unanticipated hospital admissions	0
Deep venous thrombosis	0
Mortality	0
Acute urinary retention	1
Orthostatic hypotension, treated with fluids	7
Orthostatic hypotension, treated with fluids and vasoconstrictor	3
Airway management	
Oral airway	0
Nasal airway	1
Endotracheal tube/LMA	0
Face mask with oxygen/positive pressure ventilation	7
PONV	5

Abbreviation: LMA, Laryngeal Mask Airway.

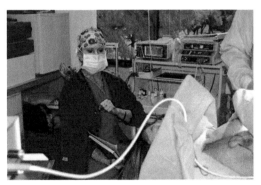

Fig. 1. Anesthesia provider directly observing patient for comfort level and airway, with electronic monitor, drugs, and anesthesia machine readily available.

determining future propofol doses. During this time, the patient also receives fentanyl, 0.5 µg/kg, and ketamine, 0.25 mg/kg, to provide a brief and mild dissociative state during the infiltration of the local anesthetic (**Table 2**, for dosages). The goal of this measured use of agents is to provide adequate sedation while maintaining spontaneous respirations and adequate oxygenation, without assistance or supplemental oxygen. A mixture (1:1) of lidocaine HCl 1% with epinephrine and bupivacaine HCl 0.25% with epinephrine local infiltration is used to provide rapid onset and long duration of the local anesthetic effect.

Painful stimuli that result in a patient response, including movement, verbal complaints, or a subtle change in breathing pattern, should be managed by infiltration of additional local anesthetic by the surgeon. A small amount of propofol may be given to relax the patient. However, when patient movement seems independent of painful stimuli, it may be positional discomfort, restlessness, or undisclosed claustrophobia. Whereas additional propofol may diminish this movement, it may also result in apnea. In the authors' experience, restlessness is best controlled with a bolus of diazepam, 5 mg, which does not result in apnea or significantly delay discharge.

PONV is a debilitating consequence of anesthesia, which leads to patient dissatisfaction and prolonged time at the surgical facility. Approaches to preventing PONV have been studied extensively with rates of nausea from 4% to 38.5% in those who were treated prophylactically and 10% to 79% without prophylaxis.[15–17] In their experience, the authors have found PONV to be uncommon, and they attribute this to decreased narcotic requirement because pain is well controlled by the long-acting local anesthetic. Chemoprophylaxis begins with the initial use of droperidol, 0.625 mg, along with midazolam, and single dose of dexamethasone, 8 to 10 mg after the first dose of propofol. The propofol should be given before the steroid to mitigate acute urethral irritation, frequently caused by dexamethasone. Ondansetron, 4 mg,

is administered intravenously within the last hour of surgery. Additionally, adequate hydration is important for PONV prevention and hemodynamic stability. A single dose of ketorolac, 30 mg, is given at the end of the procedure to provide extended pain relief (**Table 3**).

With conscious sedation, most patients meet discharge criteria when they arrive in the recovery area. However, the patient should be observed

Table 3
Medications listed by actions

Midazolam	Anxiolysis, some contemporaneous amnesia,[18,20] short duration of action
Propofol	Hypnotic, some antiemetic effects, short duration of action[18]
Fentanyl	Narcotic, blunts pain response to local injections, decreases propofol dosing needs, provides some postoperative pain control[18]
Ketamine	Dissociative, no respiratory depression at recommended doses, may decrease fentanyl and propofol requirements[19,20]
Diazepam	Skeletal muscle relaxant, antispasmodic, anxiolytic
Ketorolac	Nonnarcotic postoperative pain control
Dexamethasone	Sense of well-being postoperatively, antiemetic action,[18,22] late effect on PONV, seems to have synergistic effects when given with ondansetron[18,21]
Droperidol	Antiemetic action in CTZ and area postrema, does not alter cardiac refractory period or produce extrapyramidal effects in low dose[18,20,22] Always give with or after benzodiazepine to avoid anxiety sometimes associated with this drug[22]
Ondansetron	5-HT3 receptor antagonist, acts peripherally on vagus nerve terminals and centrally in CTZ[18,22]

Abbreviation: CTZ, Chemoreceptor Trigger Zone in the area postrema.

Table 2
Conscious sedation dosing regimen

	Initial Dose	Follow-Up Dose
Midazolam	0.025 mg/kg	0.025–0.04 mg/kg
Propofol	0.4–0.7 mg/kg	0.3–0.5 mg/kg
Fentanyl	0.4–0.7 µg/kg	0.6–1 µg/kg
Ketamine	0.15–0.3 mg/kg	0.15–0.3 mg/kg
Diazepam	NA	0.05–0.07 mg/kg

and monitored until vital signs and level of consciousness are appropriate for discharge. Because the surgical area is anesthetized locally to permit surgery, early postoperative pain management is simplified, reducing the use of narcotics or other analgesics that prolong recovery and increase the risk of PONV.

DISCUSSION ON CONSCIOUS SEDATION FROM VARIOUS PERSPECTIVES
Patient Selection

Patient selection is essential to the success of this technique. The patient should be healthy, ASA I or II, relatively mature, and emotionally stable. However, children typically respond well to conscious sedation. Any patient who has anxiety tendencies, claustrophobia, or a previous unsatisfactory experience with a procedure done under sedation should be counseled thoroughly before offered this approach. In the authors' experience, males may be more difficult patients because they may show agitation with conscious sedation.

The patient should be thoroughly informed about the method and goals of this type of anesthesia, as contrasted with a general anesthesia. The authors have found that a well-motivated, adequately prepared patient requires no premedication and can even walk from the preoperative area to the office OR. Most of the authors' patients meet or nearly meet discharge criteria at the end of the procedure and are comfortably transported to the postoperative (recovery) area in a wheelchair. The average patient is discharged from the post-surgical observation area within 20 to 30 minutes.

In the authors' experience, a wide range of cases have been successfully done in an OBS setting using local anesthesia and conscious sedation, including aesthetic facial and breast surgery and bodying contouring, including liposuction and abdominoplasty. Multiple procedures have been successfully performed under conscious sedation, but longer and more extensive combined procedures may be more appropriately done under a general anesthetic.

The Surgeon

Success with conscious sedation requires a commitment by the surgeon to exercise patience, use gentle surgical technique, and to be willing to communicate with the patient and anesthesia provider during the procedure. A surgeon experienced in the use of local anesthesia/conscious sedation develops a level of comfort by being constantly aware of the status of the patient's comfort. The surgeon must be adept at the use of local anesthesia and anesthetic wetting solutions to provide profound, effective anesthesia. Sufficient time should be allowed after the administration of the local anesthetic to provide maximum anesthesia and vasoconstriction. Should the patient experience pain during the procedure, the surgeon must pause and add additional local anesthetic, in coordination with the anesthesia provider. It is imperative that the surgeon and anesthesia provider understand that the anesthesia provider's goal is to sedate the patient, whereas the surgeon's responsibility is to provide analgesia.

The OR Nursing Staff

Although the professional activities and responsibilities of the nursing staff are independent of the type of anesthesia, conscious sedation requires certain additional considerations. All aspects of patient comfort must be considered in the "awake" patient with a prompt response to any verbal request. The entire team should avoid using alarming terminology, such as pain, knife, blood, needle, and so forth, and instead substitute such terms as discomfort, #15 (scalpel blade), drainage, and attachment (needles are attached to suture). In general in the OR, but especially with the "awake" patient, inappropriate and unnecessary conversation should be avoided. OR music should not be loud or distracting, but should be background music, of a genre selected with consideration of the patient and OR staff.

The Anesthesia Provider

In many ways, conscious sedation is more demanding of the anesthesia provider than general anesthesia, in comparable patients and surgical procedures. Because the level of sedation with propofol may unexpectedly deepen, requiring emergent airway management, the anesthesia provider must be vigilant and responsive. The administration of conscious sedation requires the anesthesia provider's constant and undivided attention, clinical expertise, and a great deal of patience.

SUMMARY

Conscious sedation is almost as much an art as it is a science, and requires the commitment of the entire OR team. It is not the easiest approach, but has several significant advantages, including safety, shorter recovery period, less nausea and vomiting, and generally a better patient experience. Also, it lends itself to OBS because it requires less space, equipment, and personnel. Low-dose propofol, along with other drugs, is the ideal agent because it provides sedation, anxiolyis, and amnesia, with rapid onset and a short duration of action. The technique described in this article includes the use of low-dose propofol with midazolam and often small doses of fentanyl, without supplemental oxygen or airway devices, or endotracheal intubation. A total of 1400 cases were reported with negligible complications, and no hospitalizations or fatalities.

REFERENCES

1. Keyes GR, Singer R, Iverson RE, et al. Mortality in outpatient surgery. Plast Reconstr Surg 2008;122:245.
2. Morello DC, Colon GA, Fredricks S, et al. Patient safety in accredited office surgical facilities. Plast Reconstr Surg 1997;99:1496.
3. Byrd HS, Barton FE, Orenstein HH, et al. Safety and efficacy in an accredited outpatient plastic surgery facility: a review of 5316 consecutive cases. Plast Reconstr Surg 2003;112:636.
4. Mustoe TA, Kim P, Schierle CF. Out patient abdominoplasty under conscious sedation. Aesthet Surg J 2007;27:442.
5. Marik PE. Propofol: therapeutic indications and side-effects. Curr Pharm Des 2004;10:3639–49.
6. Hansen KC, Samartzis D, Casas LA. An outcome study comparing intravenous sedation with midazolam/fentanyl (conscious sedation) versus propofol infusion (deep sedation) for aesthetic surgery. Plast Reconstr Surg 2003;112:1683.
7. Minutes ASA House of Delegates, Continuum of Depth of Sedation Definition of General Anesthesia and Levels of Sedation/Analgesia, October 13, 1999 and amended October 27, 2004.
8. Pollock H. Operating room fires. Plast Reconstr Surg 2009;123(1):431 [author reply: 431–2].
9. Stemp L. Etiology of hypoximia often overlooked. APSF Newsletter 2004;19(3):38–9.
10. Kryger ZB, Fine NA, Mustoe TA. The outcome of abdominoplasty performed under conscious sedation: six-year experience in 153 consecutive cases. Plast Reconstr Surg 2004;113:1807–17.
11. Yoon HD, Yoon ES, Dhong ES, et al. Low-dose propofol infusion for sedation during local anesthesia. Plast Reconstr Surg 2002;109:956–63.
12. Engel SJ, Nikesh KP, Morrison CM, et al. Operating room fires. Part II. Optimizing safety. Plast Reconstr Surg 2012;130:681–9.
13. Marcus JR, Few JW, Fine NA, et al. Optimzation of conscious sedation in plastic surgery. Plast Reconstr Surg 1999;104:1338–13845.
14. Bitar G, Mullis W, Jacobs W, et al. Safety and efficacy of office based surgery with monitored anesthesia care/sedation in 4778 consecutive plastic surgery procedures. Plast Reconstr Surg 2003;111:150–6.
15. Apfel C, Laara E, Koivuranta M, et al. A simplified risk score for predicting postoperative nausea and vomiting: conclusions from cross-validations between two centers. Anesthesiology 1999;91(3):693.
16. Tang J, Chen X, White P, et al. Antiemetic prophylaxis for office-based surgery: are the 5-HT3 receptor antagonists beneficial? Anesthesiology 2003;98(2):293–8.
17. Rajerva V, Bhardwaj N, Batra YK, et al. Comparison of ondansetron with ondansetron and dexamethasone in prevention of PONV in diagnostic laparoscopy. Can J Anaesth 1999;46(1):40–4.
18. Marco AP. Understanding Ambulatory Anesthetics. Supplement to OutPatient Magazine 2005;8–15.
19. Courtney B. Ketamine: a new look at an old drug. Curr Rev Nurse Anesth 2009;32(14):165–76.
20. Deng XM, Xiao WJ, Lou MP, et al. The use of midazolam and small dose ketamine for sedation and analgesia during local anesthesia. Anesth Analg 2001;93:1174–7.
21. Gan TJ, Meyer TA, Apfel CC, et al. Antiemetic therapy for PONV prophylaxis. Anesth Analg 2003;97:6271.
22. Rodriquez Y, Candiotti K. Current Review on Postoperative Nausea and Vomiting (PONV). Curr Rev Nurse Anesth 2009;32(4):37–52.

Deep Venous Thrombosis
Prevention and Management

Ronald E. Iverson, MD[a,b,*], Janet L. Gomez, RN, BA, RNFA[c]

KEYWORDS

- Deep vein thrombosis • Patient safety • Postoperative complications
- Postoperative risk assessment • Pulmonary emboli • Venous thromboembolism

KEY POINTS

- Deep vein thrombosis and its possible sequela of pulmonary embolism are a major risk for plastic surgery patients.
- Patients undergoing an abdominoplasty are at a significant risk of death due to pulmonary emboli.
- Risk assessment is the basis for prevention of thromboembolic phenomena.
- Measures to prevent deep venous thrombosis must be taken based on risk stratification.
- Early diagnosis and treatment of deep venous thrombosis or pulmonary emboli are essential to decrease the risks of these serious sequelae.

The incidence of thromboembolic phenomena, including deep venous thrombosis (DVT) and its feared sequela of pulmonary embolism (PE), are major health care issues and known postoperative risks of lengthy surgical procedures.[1,2] *The Surgeon General's Call to Action to Prevent Deep Vein Thrombosis and Pulmonary Embolism*, 2008 estimated that 350,000 to 600,000 Americans suffer annually from DVT and PE and that at least 100,000 deaths per year may be related to these diseases.[3] In 2009, the National Quality Forum had even more impressive statistics[4]: each year more than 900,000 Americans form DVTs, of which 500,000 experience a PE, resulting in roughly 300,000 deaths. Surgeons who operate in ambulatory facilities must become aware of these health risks for their patients.

Overview

An historical review of the plastic surgery literature reveals studies that offer recommendations for both DVT prophylaxis and risk management, starting with a 1999 article by Noel McDevitt.[5] The executive committee of the American Society of Plastic Surgeons (ASPS)–approved *Venous Thromboembolism Task Force Report* identified the best practices for DVT/PE prevention and treatment.[6] The ASPS Task Force on Patient Safety has also published articles offering recommendations for DVT prophylaxis based on levels of risk in ambulatory surgery settings.[7–9] The need for awareness of DVT/PE prophylaxis in plastic surgery, and specifically in liposuction and abdominoplasty procedures, has been the basis for numerous articles.[9–18] The correlation of DVT/PE and body-contouring surgery after massive weight loss was addressed by Kenkel,[19] for abdominal contouring by Hatef and colleagues,[20,21] and is still receiving attention as documented by Egrari[21] in 2012. The risk of DVT is even greater in patients receiving orthopedic care and in certain categories of trauma and general surgery than in plastic surgery. There is extensive published literature to support this conclusion.[22–29]

Facelifts and their association with DVT/PE were documented by Rigg[30] and by Reinisch and colleagues[31] in 1998, and still remain an important

[a] Stanford University Medical School, Palo Alto, CA, USA; [b] American Association for the Accreditation of Surgical Facilities, IL, USA; [c] Ronald E. Iverson, MD, FACS, The Plastic Surgery Center, 1387 Santa Rita Road, Pleasanton, CA 94566, USA
* Corresponding author. The Plastic Surgery Center, 1387 Santa Rita Road, Pleasanton, CA 94566, USA.
E-mail address: reiversonmd@sbcglobal.net

Clin Plastic Surg 40 (2013) 389–398
http://dx.doi.org/10.1016/j.cps.2013.04.002

topic, as pointed out in the article by Abboushi and colleagues[32] in 2012. The facelift procedures that were complicated by postoperative DVT were performed under both local anesthesia with sedation and general anesthesia, continuing a long discussion as to whether avoidance of general anesthesia can decrease or eliminate DVT/PE.[33–37] Hoefflin[38] countered by reporting no major complications in 23,000 cases under general anesthesia.

AMERICAN ASSOCIATION FOR THE ACCREDITATION OF SURGICAL FACILITIES
Peer Review Data: September 2012

The American Association for the Accreditation of Surgical Facilities (AAAASF), through its quality assurance and peer review process, has previously reported on significant issues in ambulatory surgery.[14,15] The latest data are shown in **Table 1** and confirm the many reports that DVT/PE is a major problem for patients having plastic surgery. Of the 3,922,202 plastic surgery cases, there were 215 DVTs and 264 PEs for a total of 479. This is an incidence by case of 0.01222% or 1 in every 8188 cases. The largest number of venous thromboembolism (VTE), 308, occurred with abdominoplasties. The abdominoplasty procedures performed alone were 98; abdominoplasties plus 1 additional procedure were 137; plus 2 additional procedures, 58; and plus 3 additional procedures, 15, which is an incidence of 0.0666% or 1 in every 1502 cases. Total abdominoplasties that were associated with a PE were 185, with an incidence of 0.04% or 1 in every 2500 cases. The distribution of PE cases associated with abdominoplasty alone or abdominoplasties with multiple procedures is similar to the data for patients having VTE/PE. There is no significant statistical difference for VTE or PE whether the abdominoplasty is performed alone or with multiple other procedures. It has been reported in the literature that performing multiple procedures at the same time increases the risk of complications, such as VTE. These peer-reviewed data do not support that conclusion.

There were 94 deaths associated with plastic surgery, or an incidence of 0.0024% or 1 in every 41,726 cases. The incidence of death in plastic surgery procedures is 0.0017% or 1 in every 58,779 procedures. The death rate in plastic surgery by case or procedure is less than when all specialties are combined; the number of deaths related to PE in the plastic surgery cases was 40 of 94, or 43%. It is significant that, of the 40 deaths in plastic surgery procedures, an incidence of 0.0010% or 1 in every 98,055 cases, 26 occurred with abdominoplasties for an incidence of 0.0056% or 1 in every 17,791 cases. The data also reveal that PEs have occurred with a significant number of other procedures; 5 in facelift and blepharoplasty, 5 with liposuction, 2 with buttocks/thigh extremity lift, and 2 with breast surgery.

Risk Assessment

Plastic surgery continues to emphasize risk assessment and risk-stratifying models for DVT as a basis for prevention and avoidance.[2,5,7] Many patient characteristics, behaviors, and medical histories identify increased risks for postoperative DVT. Obstetric history is important and frequently overlooked.[23] Past obstetric complications including a still birth, miscarriage, or premature birth with toxemia may indicate a serious thrombophilia defect. Postmenopausal hormone therapy and selective estrogen-receptor modulators (tamoxifen and raloxifene) are associated with 2-fold to 3-fold increased risk of venous thrombosis.[39] The factors that predisposed a patient to thrombosis or embolism in 2002 formed a limited list.[7] It has not only been expanded but better defined by Caprini and others.[22–24,40]

The 2005 Caprini Risk Assessment Model (**Fig. 1**) and its subsequent, more developed, version, the 2010 Caprini Risk Assessment Model (**Fig. 2**), are thorough, noting common risk factors for DVT and PE. Each factor is weighted 1, 2, 3, or 5 points, depending on its significance for risk. An overall total risk category score is then assigned (**Table 2**). A correlation between the total risk score and proven VTE incidents in surgical patients has been reported.[24,41,42]

The assessment of postoperative VTE risk in patients having plastic surgery, using both the 2005 and 2010 Caprini Risk Assessment Models, was studied by Pannucci and colleagues.[43] Their conclusion identified the 2005 Caprini model as a more appropriate method for risk stratification of patients having plastic surgery than the 2010 model.

Although the Caprini assessment models do not include smoking as a risk factor, the presence of coagulation abnormalities associated with smoking[44] may further increase the risk for DVT/PE. Tobacco smoking has been associated with increased serum homocysteine, representing a 3-point risk factor in the model. The interrelationship between smoking, its procoagulant mechanisms, and VTE awaits further therapeutic studies. The importance of evidence-based medicine in these areas mandates further research.[45–47]

Prevention

The strategies for prevention of DVT/PE are extensive and most often based on preoperative risk

Table 1
American association for the accreditation of surgical facilities, plastic surgery data for VTE, PE, and deaths (September 2012)

Total Cases all AAAASF Specialties	5,416,071				
Total Procedures all AAAASF Specialties	7,629,686	1.41	Procedures per Case		
Plastic Surgery Cases	3,922,202				
Plastic Surgery Procedures	5,525,255	1.41	Procedures per Case		
		Incidence % by Case	1 in # Case	Incidence % by Procedure	1 in # Procedure
All Deaths all Specialties	184	0.0034%	29,435	0.0024%	41,466
		Incidence % by Plastic Surgery Case	1 in # Plastic Surgery Case	Incidence % by Plastic Surgery Procedure	1 in # Plastic Surgery Procedure
All Plastic Surgery Deaths	94	0.0024%	41,726	0.0017%	58,779
Total Abdominoplasties Performed	462,564				
Abdominoplasty Alone	176,092				
Abdominoplasty + 1 other procedure	187,847				
Abdominoplasty + 2 other procedures	73,869				
Abdominoplasty + 3 other procedures	24,756				
		Incidence % by Case	1 in # Case	Incidence % by Procedure	1 in # Procedure
Total Plastic Surgery VTE	479	0.0122%	8188	0.0087%	11,535
Plastic Surgery DVT	215	0.0055%	18,243	0.0039%	25,699
Plastic Surgery PE	264	0.0048%	20,929	0.0048%	20,929
		Incidence % by Case	1 in # Case		
Abdominoplasty + VTE	308	0.0666%	1502		
VTE Abdominoplasty Alone	98	0.0557%	1797		
VTE Abdominoplasty + 1 other procedure	137	0.0729%	1371		
VTE Abdominoplasty + 2 other procedures	58	0.0785%	1274		
VTE Abdominoplasty + 3 other procedures	15	0.0606%	1650		
		Incidence % by Case	1 in # Case		
Abdominoplasty + PE	185	0.0400%	2500		
PE Abdominoplasty Alone	60	0.0341%	2935		
PE Abdominoplasty + 1 other procedure	81	0.0431%	2319		
PE Abdominoplasty + 2 other procedures	37	0.0501%	1996		

(continued on next page)

Table 1
(continued)

		Incidence % by Case	1 in # Case	Incidence % by Procedure	1 in # Procedure
PE Abdominoplasty + 3 other procedures	7	0.0283%	3537		
Deaths PE All Plastic Surgery Procedures	40	0.0010%	98,055	0.0007%	138,131
Deaths PE Abdominoplasty Alone	6	0.0034%	29,349		
Deaths PE Abdominoplasty + 1 other procedure	10	0.0053%	18,785		
Deaths PE Abdominoplasty + 2 other procedure	9	0.0122%	8208		
Deaths PE Abdominoplasty + 3 other procedure	1	0.0040%	24,756		
Total Deaths PE Abdominoplasty	26	0.0056%	17,791		
Deaths Facelift and Blepharoplasty	5				
Deaths PE Liposuction	5				
Death PE Buttocks Thigh Extremity Lift	2				
Deaths PE Breast Augmentation or Lift	2				

Data from American Association for Ambulatory Surgical Facilities, Inc. Internet Based Quality Assurance and Peer Review Program. Available at: http://www.aaaasf.org.

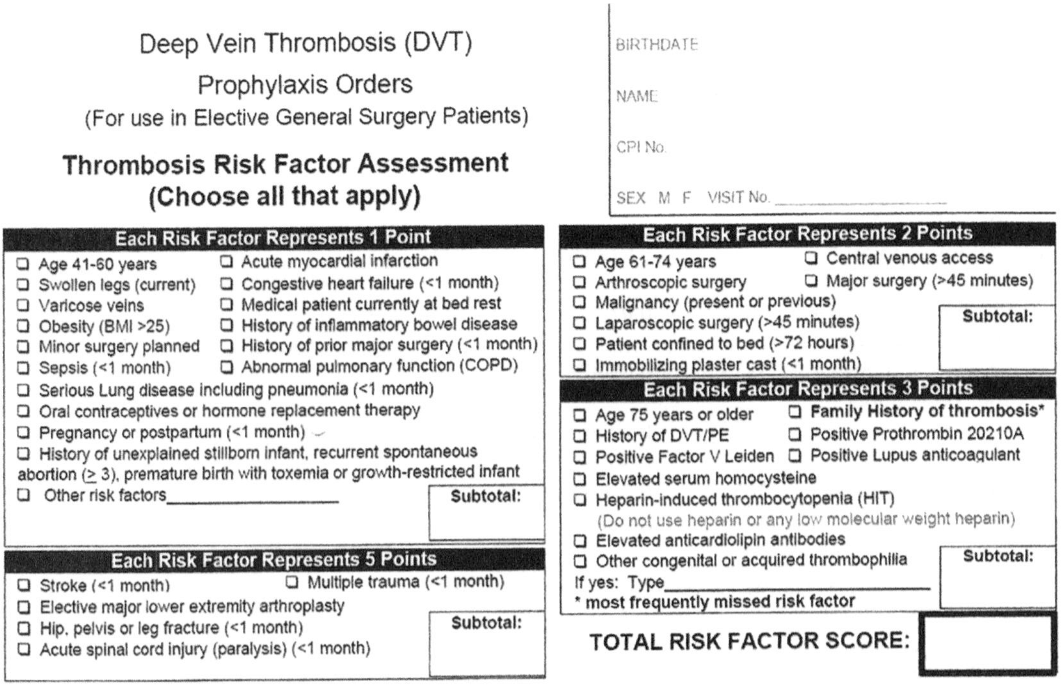

Deep Vein Thrombosis (DVT)

Prophylaxis Orders

(For use in Elective General Surgery Patients)

Thrombosis Risk Factor Assessment (Choose all that apply)

BIRTHDATE

NAME

CPI No.

SEX M F VISIT No. _____

Each Risk Factor Represents 1 Point

- ☐ Age 41-60 years
- ☐ Acute myocardial infarction
- ☐ Swollen legs (current)
- ☐ Congestive heart failure (<1 month)
- ☐ Varicose veins
- ☐ Medical patient currently at bed rest
- ☐ Obesity (BMI >25)
- ☐ History of inflammatory bowel disease
- ☐ Minor surgery planned
- ☐ History of prior major surgery (<1 month)
- ☐ Sepsis (<1 month)
- ☐ Abnormal pulmonary function (COPD)
- ☐ Serious Lung disease including pneumonia (<1 month)
- ☐ Oral contraceptives or hormone replacement therapy
- ☐ Pregnancy or postpartum (<1 month)
- ☐ History of unexplained stillborn infant, recurrent spontaneous abortion (≥ 3), premature birth with toxemia or growth-restricted infant
- ☐ Other risk factors_____

Subtotal:

Each Risk Factor Represents 5 Points

- ☐ Stroke (<1 month)
- ☐ Multiple trauma (<1 month)
- ☐ Elective major lower extremity arthroplasty
- ☐ Hip, pelvis or leg fracture (<1 month)
- ☐ Acute spinal cord injury (paralysis) (<1 month)

Subtotal:

Each Risk Factor Represents 2 Points

- ☐ Age 61-74 years
- ☐ Central venous access
- ☐ Arthroscopic surgery
- ☐ Major surgery (>45 minutes)
- ☐ Malignancy (present or previous)
- ☐ Laparoscopic surgery (>45 minutes)
- ☐ Patient confined to bed (>72 hours)
- ☐ Immobilizing plaster cast (<1 month)

Subtotal:

Each Risk Factor Represents 3 Points

- ☐ Age 75 years or older
- ☐ Family History of thrombosis*
- ☐ History of DVT/PE
- ☐ Positive Prothrombin 20210A
- ☐ Positive Factor V Leiden
- ☐ Positive Lupus anticoagulant
- ☐ Elevated serum homocysteine
- ☐ Heparin-induced thrombocytopenia (HIT)
  (Do not use heparin or any low molecular weight heparin)
- ☐ Elevated anticardiolipin antibodies
- ☐ Other congenital or acquired thrombophilia
If yes: Type_____
* most frequently missed risk factor

Subtotal:

TOTAL RISK FACTOR SCORE:

Fig. 1. The 2005 Caprini Risk Assessment Model. COPD, chronic obstructive pulmonary disease. (*Adapted from* Caprini JA. Thrombosis risk assessment as a guide to quality patient care. Dis Mon 2005;51:70–8; with permission.)

CHOOSE ALL THAT APPLY

A1: Each Risk Factor Represents 1 Point
O Age 40-59 years
O Minor surgery planned
O History of prior major surgery
O Varicose veins
O History of inflammatory bowel disease
O Swollen legs (current)
O Obesity (BMI > 30)
O Acute myocardial infarction (<l month)
O Congestive heart failure (< 1 month)
O Sepsis (< 1 month)
O Serious lung disease incl. pneumonia (< 1 month)
O Abnormal pulmonary function (Chronic obstructive pulmonary disease)
O Medical patient currently at bed rest
O Leg plaster cast or brace
O Central venous access
O Blood transfusion (< 1 month)
O Other risk factor/s_____ _____

B: Each Risk Factor Represents 2 Points
O Age 60-74 years
O Major surgery (> 60 minutes)*
O Arthroscopic surgery (> 60 minutes)*
O Laparoscopic surgery (> 60 minutes)*
O Previous malignancy
O Morbid obesity (BMI > 40)

C: Each Risk Factor Represents 3 Points
O Age 75 years or more
O Major surgery lasting 2-3 hours*
O BMI > 50 (venous stasis syndrome)
O History of SVT, DVT/PE
O **Family history of DVT/PE**
O Present cancer or chemotherapy
O Positive Factor V Leiden
O Positive Prothrombin 20210A
O Elevated serum homocysteine
O Positive Lupus anticoagulant
O Elevated anticardiolipin antibodies
O Heparin-induced thrombocytopenia (HIT)
O Other thrombophilia- Type_____

A2: For Women Only (Each Represents 1 Point)
O Oral contraceptives or hormone replacement therapy
O Pregnancy or postpartum (<1 month)
O History of unexplained stillborn infant, recurrent spontaneous abortion (≥ 3), premature birth with toxemia of pregnancy or growth restricted infant

D: Each Risk Factor Represents 5 Points
O Elective major lower extremity arthroplasty
O Hip, pelvis or leg fracture (< 1 month)
O Stroke (< 1 month)
O Multiple trauma (< 1 month)
O Acute spinal cord injury (paralysis)(< 1month)
O Major surgery lasting over 3 hours*

TOTAL RISK FACTOR SCORE:

Fig. 2. The 2010 Caprini Risk Assessment Model. BMI, body mass index; DVT/PE, deep venous thrombosis/pulmonary embolus; SVT, superficial venous thrombophlebitis. (*Adapted from* Caprini JA. Risk assessment as a guide to thrombosis prophylaxis. Curr Opin Pulm Med 2010;16:448–52; with permission.)

Table 2
Risk assessment categories. The 2005 Caprini Risk Assessment Model

Risk Factor Score	Risk Level
0–1	Low risk
2	Moderate risk
3–4	High risk
5 or more	Highest risk

Adapted from Caprini JA. Thrombosis risk assessment as a guide to quality patient care. Dis Mon 2005;51:70–8; with permission.

assessment for DVT.[11,23–25,40] For instance, the patient's risk factors for increased bleeding are critical to evaluate because the presence of these factors may rule out the use of chemoprophylaxis. Risk factors for increased bleeding are listed in **Box 1**.

It is also important to identify and appraise any relevant findings before intermittent pneumatic compression (IPC) devices are automatically used. Peripheral arterial disease, congestive heart failure, acute superficial venous thrombophlebitis, or DVT are known diseases and conditions that are contraindicated for IPC therapy.

Box 1
Risk factors for increased bleeding

- Current medications such as aspirin or Coumadin
- Family history of bleeding disorder
- History of heparin-induced thrombocytopenia
- Known acquired bleeding disorder
- Patient bruises or swells easily
- Platelet count less than 100,000/mm^3
- Previous bleeding issues during surgery or dental procedures

---

The prophylaxis regime,[1,23–25] based on the Caprini Risk Assessment Model, is shown in **Table 3**. The basic recommendations in this table should be augmented with a comprehensive perioperative and intraoperative approach.[1,10,20,48,49] The use of chemoprophylaxis as part of the approach to prevention is explained in the article by Alan Gold, MD, elsewhere in this issue.

Somogyi and colleagues[49] thought that their preventative approach lowered the risk of VTE in abdominoplasties to a level that made chemoprophylaxis unnecessary. They made numerous recommendations, but the most significant seem to

be (1) celecoxib (Celebrex) 200 mg, taken 1 hour before surgery, (2) use of graded compression stockings beginning 24 hours before surgery, (3) IPC devices in place before surgery and maintained until discharge from the postanesthesia care unit, (4) maintenance of normothermia, and (5) encouraging ambulation as early as possible. Surgical time was minimized by their technique and staff training. These suggestions are reasonable and should be proactively considered to improve patient safety.

The authors use and recommend the strategies listed in **Box 2** for postoperative management of surgical patients.

The current standard for IPC devices from the AAAASF, Version 13 200.017.030, states that sequential compression devices are used for surgical procedures of 1 hour or longer, except for procedures performed under local anesthesia.[50] This reasonable recommendation should be adhered to no matter what level of risk is identified for the patient, unless the contraindications previously discussed are present.

Seruya and colleagues[1] found that the incidence of treated patients who present with high-risk factors for DVT are sizable and comprise 15% of the population of patients having plastic surgery. His studies suggest that thromboprophylaxis is more effective in this highest risk factor group than mechanical prophylaxis alone. All these risk factors and risk levels must be discussed with individual patients before the determination of their candidacy for surgery; this discussion is an essential part of an adequate informed consent. The patient's decision to have surgery and the surgeon's decision to perform surgery hinge on those factors and levels of risks. Patients who are in the highest risk category, especially if that risk is double digit, may need to forego elective quality-of-life procedures given that their total risk factor score indicates an extremely high risk of DVT/PE.

Table 3
Prophylaxis regime. The 2010 Caprini Risk Assessment Model

Total Risk Factor Scores	Risk Level	Prophylaxis Regime
0–1	Low	Early ambulation
2	Moderate	ES or IPC or LDUH or LMWH
3–4	High	IPC or LDUH or LMWH alone or in combination with ES or IPC
5 or more	Highest	Pharmacologic: LDUH, LMWH, warfarin or FAC Xa alone or in combination with ES or IPC

Abbreviations: ES, elastic stocking; FAC Xa, factor, X inhibitor; IPC, pneumatic impression device; LDUH, low-dose unfractionated heparin; LMWH, low-molecular-weight heparin.

Adapted from Caprini JA. Risk assessment as a guide to thrombosis prophylaxis. Curr Opin Pulm Med 2010;16:448–52; with permission.

Box 2
Prevention through postoperative patient management

- Ambulation every hour
- Avoid popliteal pressure while sitting
- Foot elevation and flexion exercises at rest
- Graded compression elastic stockings for 7 days
- Hydration
- Smoking cessation

Diagnosis

DVT, in itself, is not likely to be fatal. One-half of affected patients have an asymptomatic presentation so that its diagnosis requires confirmatory laboratory tests such as duplex ultrasound (US) imaging or contrast phlebography.[24] However, the frequently associated sequela of a PE has a high mortality. DVT is historically associated with the Virchow triad of venous stasis, vascular injury, and hypercoagulability. DVT can present with the vague symptoms of feeling dizzy and faint or present dramatically with a severely swollen leg, sometimes discolored white or blue.

The early diagnosis of DVT is vital to prevent untoward sequelae from the thrombosis in the leg and to prevent a possible resulting PE. DVT most commonly develops in the veins of the calf muscle and has a low incidence of clinically significant emboli if it remains within the calf area. However, without appropriate treatment, 20% of venous thrombi in the calf propagate and pose a serious threat. At least 50% of proximal deep venous thrombi are associated with PE or recurrent DVT.[10]

Awareness and knowledge of the symptoms of DVT and associated VTE are critical for all individuals involved in postoperative communications and care with the ambulatory surgical patient. Every office staff member, from the secretary answering the patient's calls to the nursing staff providing postoperative advice and care, must be trained to recognize the sometimes vague complaints that may indicate the presence of the disease. These complaints are listed in **Box 3**.

When in doubt, and in the absence of the surgeon, staff members should instruct any postoperative patient, even those who present with symptoms 3 to 6 months after the procedure, to seek medical care immediately. Any patient contacting the office with complaints of cardiac or respiratory distress should be directed to contact emergency medical services for transport to the emergency room for a physician's evaluation. These symptoms are listed in **Box 4**.

The ninth edition of *The American College of Chest Physicians Evidence-based Clinical Practice Guidelines* on thrombotic therapy and prevention of thrombosis provides multiple levels of evaluation for patients at risk for DVT.[51] In the patient with low pretest probability of first lower extremity DVT, the following tests are recommended: (1) a moderately sensitive D-dimer, (2) a highly sensitive D-dimer, or (3) compression US (CUS) of the proximal veins. If the D-dimer is positive, further testing with CUS of the proximal veins rather than whole-leg US or venography is advised. If the CUS of the proximal veins is positive, it is recommended that confirmatory venography is performed instead of instituting treatment of DVT.

For the patient with high pretest probability of first lower extremity DVT, proximal CUS or whole-leg US is recommended. If the proximal CUS or whole-leg US is positive for DVT, treatment is recommended rather than confirmatory venography. In patients with high pretest probability, the moderately or highly sensitive D-dimer should not be used as a stand-alone test to rule out DVT. The whole-leg US may be preferred to proximal CUS in patients unable to return for serial testing and in those with severe symptoms consistent with calf DVT or risk factors for extensive distal DVT.

In patients with suspected lower extremity DVT in whom US is impractical, for example in a case in which there is excessive fluid or subcutaneous tissue to prevent adequate assessment of compressibility or diagnosis, computed tomography venography is suggested. Magnetic resonance (MR) venography or MR direct thrombus imaging

---

Box 3
Manifestations of DVT or PE that may elicit calls to the office

- Chest pain
- Fainting
- Feeling dizzy, or faint leg color change
- Leg pain
- Leg swelling
- Leg tenderness
- Shortness of breath or tachypnea

Box 4
Manifestations of DVT or PE requiring a physician's evaluation

- Hemoptysis
- Transient or orthostatic hypotension
- Transient hypoxemia
- Unexplained decrease in level of consciousness
- Suspected postoperative myocardial infarction
- Postoperative nonhemorrhagic stroke
- Postoperative pneumonia
- Unexplained sudden death
- Venous engorgement of the leg

can be used as an alternative to venography. Patients suspected of DVT may choose treatment rather than venography.

Treatment

Once the diagnosis of DVT is made, the surgeon must immediately consider a consultation with the appropriate medical physician specialist and possibly a vascular surgeon. Without appropriate treatment, 20% of calf vein thrombi propagate proximately to where they pose a serious threat. At least 50% of proximal DVTs are associated with a PE or recurrent DVT, 10% were immediately fatal with PE, and 5% caused death later as a result of right ventricular dysfunction and/or pulmonary hypertension.[10] The other major problem following a DVT is postthrombotic syndrome (PTS).[25,26] PTS is clinically associated with leg pain, swelling of the leg, and varicose veins.

The protocol for antithrombotic therapy is covered in the 2012 The American College of Chest Physicians Evidence-based Clinical Practice Guidelines,[51] summarizing bodies of evidence to offer 600 recommendations for diagnosing, preventing, and treating DVT. The guidelines suggest that the initial anticoagulation for acute DVT be a parenteral anticoagulation low-molecular-weight heparin (Enoxaparin), fondaparinux (Arixtra), intravenous unfractionated heparin, or subcutaneous heparin. This protocol is also indicated for patients with a high suspicion of acute VTE. Any patient who has been identified as high risk for bleeding dyscrasias requires special evaluation before instituting initial anticoagulation.

Catheter-directed thrombolysis must be considered because of the benefit for the prevention of the PTS. Catheter-assisted thrombus removal is also a consideration as a method of decreasing the risk of PTS and the consequences of a PE. Vena cava filters are a consideration for patients with acute proximal DVT. The inferior vena cava filter is recommended for a patient in whom anticoagulation is contraindicated.

A vitamin K antagonist is often used for the long-term treatment of DVT. Treatment considerations, like medication usage, length of treatment, and follow-up strategies, are complex issues and should be managed by an internal medicine specialist.

Discussion

Quality care measures in the health care system are at the forefront of medicine.[41] There is a national movement to make DVT/PE a so-called never event and evidence-based medicine must be applied to the evaluation of this complex problem. It seems from all current information that DVT/PE problems will never be eliminated.

The level of awareness of DVT/PE as a major cause of mortality in ambulatory surgery has dramatically increased over the past 10 years. There are many strategies for the prevention and treatment of DVT/PE. It is only through both patients and surgeons being informed about the dangers and realities of DVT that the incidence of the problem can be decreased. It is imperative that plastic surgeons continue their efforts for increased public awareness and patient education related to the risk factors and symptoms of DVT. Plastic surgeons must routinely incorporate preoperative DVT risk assessment models for all patients who are to undergo surgery as well as apply a renewed vigilance on patient selection. The prevention protocol should be based on risk assessment and all appropriate recommended perioperative and postoperative modalities for prevention must be used. Surgeon and their staff must be trained to identify and diagnose a DVT for when prevention fails. If a DVT is suspected, appropriate treatment using a specialist medical consultation is a necessity and should be instituted immediately.

When these approaches are used by all plastics surgeons, a significant improvement in patient safety and surgical outcomes should be seen. The overall safety of performing surgery in an ambulatory setting is well documented. Continued vigilance is essential for all safety issues in the surgery suite, but those precautions for DVT/PE prevention should be foremost because those diseases are frequently associated with a patient's disability and even death.

REFERENCES

1. Seruya M, Venturi ML, Iorio ML, et al. Efficacy and safety of venous thromboembolism prophylaxis in highest risk plastic surgery patients. Plast Reconstr Surg 2008;122:1701–8.
2. The Doctors Company. Deep venous thrombosis and pulmonary embolism in plastic surgery office procedures. Available at: http://www.thedoctors.com. Accessed January 30, 2006.
3. US Department of Health and Human Services. The Surgeon General's call to action to prevent deep vein thrombosis and pulmonary embolism. 2008. Available at: http://www.surgeongeneral.gov/topics/deepvein/calltoaction/call-to-action-on-dvt-2008.pdf. Accessed July 31, 2012.
4. The National Quality Forum. NQF portfolio of completed projects. 2009. Available at: http://www.qualityforum.org/pdf/IsNQFprojects%20Completed

%20Current_March2009.doc/. Accessed August 20, 2012.

5. McDevitt NB. Deep vein thrombosis prophylaxis. Plast Reconstr Surg 1999;104:1923–8.

6. Murphy RX Jr, Alderman A, Gutowski K, et al. Evidenced-based practices for thromboembolism prevention: summary of the ASPS Venous Thromboembolism Task Force report. EBM special topic-online. Plast Reconstr Surg 2012;130:259.

7. Iverson RE. ASPS Task Force: patient safety in office-based surgery facilities: I. Procedures in the office-based surgery setting. Plast Reconstr Surg 2002;110(5):1337–42.

8. Iverson RE, Lynch DJ. ASPS Task Force: patient safety in office-based surgery facilities: II. Patient selection. Plast Reconstr Surg 2002;110(7):1785–92.

9. Iverson RE, Lynch DJ. ASPS Committee on Patient Safety. Practice advisory on liposuction. Plast Reconstr Surg 2004;113(5):1478–96.

10. Boughton G, Rios JL, Rohrich RJ, et al. Deep venous thrombosis prophylaxis practice and treatment strategies among plastic surgeons: survey results. Plast Reconstr Surg 2007;119:157–74.

11. Davidson SP, Venturi ML, Attiger CE, et al. Prevention of venous thromboembolism in the plastic surgery patient. Plast Reconstr Surg 2004;114: 43e–51e.

12. Gravante G, Araco A, Sorge R, et al. Pulmonary embolism after combined abdominoplasty and flank liposuction: a correlation with the amount of fat removed. Ann Plast Surg 2008;60:604–8.

13. Iverson RE, Pao VS. Liposuction. Plast Reconstr Surg 2008;121(4):1–11.

14. Keyes GR, Singer R, Iverson RE, et al. Analysis of outpatient surgery center safety using an internet-based quality improvement and peer review program. Plast Reconstr Surg 2004;113(6): 1760–70.

15. Keyes GR, Singer R, Iverson RE, et al. Mortality in outpatient surgery. Plast Reconstr Surg 2008;122: 245–50.

16. Murphy RX Jr, Peterson EA, Adkinson JM, et al. Plastic surgeon compliance with national safety initiatives: clinical outcomes and "never events". Plast Reconstr Surg 2010;126:653–6.

17. Young VL, Watson ME. The need for venous thromboembolism (VTE) prophylaxis in plastic surgery. Aesthet Surg J 2006;26(2):157–75.

18. Gutowski KA. Commentary on: venous thromboembolism in abdominoplasty: a comprehensive approach to lower procedural risk. Aesthet Surg J 2006;32(3):330–1.

19. Kenkel JM. Body contouring surgery after massive weight loss. Plast Reconstr Surg 2006; 117(1):1S–85S.

20. Hatef DA, Trussler AP, Kenkel JM. Procedural risk for venous thromboembolism in abdominal contouring surgery: a systematic review of the literature. Aesthet Surg J 2010;125:352–62.

21. Egrari S. Outpatient-based massive weight loss body contouring: a review of 260 consecutive cases. Aesthet Surg J 2012;32(4):474–83.

22. Anderson FA Jr, Spencer FA. Risk factors for venous thromboembolism. Circulation 2003;107: 19–116.

23. Caprini JA. Thrombosis risk assessment as a guide to quality patient care. Dis Mon 2005;51:70–8.

24. Caprini JA. Risk assessment as a guide for the prevention of the many faces of venous thromboembolism. Am J Surg 2010;199(Suppl 1A):S3–10.

25. Caprini JA. Risk assessment as a guide to thrombosis prophylaxis. Curr Opin Pulm Med 2010;16: 448–52.

26. Kahn SR. The post-thrombotic syndrome: the forgotten morbidity of deep venous thrombosis. J Thromb Thrombolysis 2006;21:41–8.

27. Lopez JA, Kearon C, Lee AY. Deep venous thrombosis. Hematology Am Soc Hematol Educ Program 2004;439–56.

28. Mommertz G, Sigala F, Glowka TD, et al. Differences of venous thromboembolic risks in vascular, general, and trauma surgery patients. J Cardiovasc Surg (Torino) 2007;48:727–33.

29. Tamiriz LJ, Segal JB, Krishnan JA, et al. Usefulness of clinical prediction rules for the diagnosis of venous thromboembolism: a systematic review. Am J Med 2004;117:676–84.

30. Rigg BM. Deep vein thrombosis after face-lift surgery [letter]. Plast Reconstr Surg 1997;100:1363.

31. Reinisch JF, Bresnick SD, Walker JWT, et al. Deep venous thrombosis and pulmonary embolus after facelift: a study of incidence and prophylaxis. Plast Reconstru Surg 2001;107:1570–5.

32. Abboushi N, Yezhelyev M, Symbas J, et al. Facelift complications and the risk of venous thromboembolism: a single center's experience. Aesthet Surg J 2012;32(4):413–20.

33. Bitar G, Mullis W, Jacobs W, et al. Safety and efficacy of office-based surgery with monitored anesthesia care/sedation in 4778 consecutive plastic surgery procedures. Plast Reconstr Surg 2003; 111(1):150–6.

34. Iverson RE. Discussion of safety and efficacy of office-based surgery with monitored anesthesia care/sedation in 4778 consecutive plastic surgery cases. Plast Reconstr Surg 2003;111:1.

35. Iverson RE. Discussion: safety and efficacy of office-based surgery with monitored anesthesia care/sedation in 4778 consecutive plastic surgery cases. Plast Reconstru Surg 2003;112:645–6.

36. Byrd HS, Barton FE, Orenstein HH, et al. Safety and efficacy in an accredited outpatient plastic surgery facility: a review of 5316 consecutive cases. Plast Reconstr Surg 2003;112:636–41.

37. Singer R. Discussion: safety and efficacy in an accredited outpatient plastic surgery facility: a review of 5316 consecutive cases. Plast Reconstr Surg 2003;112:642–4.

38. Hoefflin SM, Bornstein JB, Gordon M. General anesthesia in an office-based plastic surgery facility: a report on more than 23,000 consecutive office-based procedures under general anesthesia with no significant anesthetic complications. Plast Reconstr Surg 2001;107:243.

39. Cushman M, Kuller LH, Prentice R. Estrogen plus progestin and risk of venous thrombosis. JAMA 2004;292(13):1573–80.

40. Wilkins EG, Pannucci CJ, Bailey SH, et al. Preliminary report on the PSEF Venous Thromboembolism Prevention Study (VTEPS): validation of the Caprini Risk Assessment Model in plastic and reconstructive surgery patients. Plast Reconstr Surg 2010; 126:107–8.

41. Muntz JE, Michota FA. Prevention and management of venous thromboembolism in the surgical patient: options by surgery type and individual patient risk factors. Am J Surg 2010;199(Suppl 1A): S11–20.

42. Passman MA. Mandated quality measures and economic implications of venous thromboembolism prevention and management. Am J Surg 2010;199(Suppl 1A):S21–31.

43. Pannucci CJ, Barta RJ, Protschy PR, et al. Assessment of postoperative venous thromboembolism risk in plastic surgery patients using the 2005 and 2010 Caprini risk score. Plast Reconstr Surg 2012;130:343–53.

44. Tapson VF. The role of smoking in coagulation and thromboembolism in chronic obstructive pulmonary disease. Proc Am Thorac Soc 2005;2:71–7.

45. Geerts WH, Bergqvist D, Pineo GF, et al. Prevention of venous thromboembolism: American College of Chest Physicians evidence-based clinical practice guidelines. Chest 2008;133:381s–453s.

46. Burns PB, Rohrich RJ, Chung KC. The levels of evidence and their role in evidence-based medicine. Plast Reconstr Surg 2011;128:305–10.

47. Sullivan D, Chung KC, Eaves FF III, et al. Editorial: the level of evidence pyramid: indicating levels of evidence in plastic and reconstructive surgery articles. Plast Reconstr Surg 2011;128:311–4.

48. Rohrich RJ, Rios JL. Venous thromboembolism in cosmetic plastic surgery: maximizing patient safety. Plast Reconstr Surg 2003;112:871–2.

49. Somogyi RB, Ahmad J, Shih JG, et al. Venous thromboembolism in abdominoplasty: a comprehensive approach to lower procedural risk. Aesthet Surg J 2011;32(3):322–9.

50. American Association for Accreditation of Ambulatory Surgery Facilities, Inc. Regular standards and checklist for accreditation of ambulatory surgery facilities, version 13, August 2011. Available at: http:// www.ironworks.us.com/asfall/PDFs%20Common/ ASF%20ASC%20Standards%20and%20Checklist %20-%20Regular.pdf. Accessed August 2, 2012.

51. Guyatt GH, Akl EA, Crowther M, et al. Executive summary: antithrombotic therapy and prevention of thrombosis, 9th edition: American college of chest physicians evidence-based clinical practice guidelines. Chest 2012;141(Suppl 2):7s–47s.

Deep Vein Thrombosis Chemoprophylaxis in Plastic Surgery

Alan Gold, MD

KEYWORDS

- Deep vein thrombosis • Chemoprophylaxis • Plastic surgery • Risk stratification

KEY POINTS

- The practice of plastic surgery is a unique mixture of art and science, and both must be carefully balanced to provide the best possible care for patients.
- Clinicians should ideally be practicing evidence-based medicine to help clinicians predict whether a treatment will do more good than harm.
- Until evidence-based medicine best-practice recommendations can be developed, it would be prudent for clinicians to empirically select, and consistently apply, a risk stratification system and prophylaxis regimen of their choice for the benefit of their patients.

INTRODUCTION

The article by Iverson and Gomez elsewhere in this issue appropriately emphasizes the prevalence of deep vein thrombosis (DVT) and the importance of its prevention and recognition in patients having plastic surgery. DVT is such a significant, but poorly appreciated, health care issue that the US Public Health Service underscored its importance in *The Surgeon General's Call to Action to Prevent Deep Vein Thrombosis and Pulmonary Embolism*, which it published in 2008.[1] It is estimated that approximately 2 million cases of DVT occur in the United States annually,[2,3] and that from 350,000 to 600,000 of those cases result in pulmonary embolus (PE),[1] with 100,000[1] to 200,000[2,3] attributable deaths. An additional undetermined number of deaths may be attributed to nonhemorrhagic stroke in association with a nonfunctioning patent foramen ovale allowing passage of thrombus.[4,5] The local signs and symptoms of DVT are caused by obstruction of venous outflow by thrombi, causing inflammation of the vein wall and inflammation and tenderness of the tissue surrounding the vein even before embolization into the pulmonary circulation.[6] It is significant that approximately 50% or more of the DVT cases are silent, offering no early clinical signs or symptoms as warning.[7,8] For those who survive the episode of DVT without those early clinical sign or symptoms, postthrombotic syndrome may also develop with significant long-term medical consequences.[9]

From the numerous, well-documented reports in the literature, it is clear that DVT, silent or not, can be a significant problem in patients having plastic surgery. What is not so clear is what should be done about it. Several approaches to DVT prophylaxis are available and, despite suggested risk assessment algorithms, who should receive what treatment or combination of treatments has not been universally accepted across this specialty. The most recent and authoritative plastic surgery publication seeking to clarify this complex issue was the report from the American Society of Plastic Surgeons' (ASPS) Venous Thromboembolism Task Force, *Evidence-based Practices for Thromboembolism Prevention*, which was approved by

Aesthetic Plastic Surgery & Cosmetic Medicine, Great Neck, NY, USA
E-mail address: ahgmd@mindspring.com

Clin Plastic Surg 40 (2013) 399–404
http://dx.doi.org/10.1016/j.cps.2013.04.003
0094-1298/13/$ – see front matter © 2013 Elsevier Inc. All rights reserved.

the ASPS Executive Committee for publication in July 2011. In conclusion, the report made the following recommendation:

Based upon the types of cases included in the literature review, Task Force members agreed that there was not enough evidence to make all-inclusive recommendations for plastic surgery prophylaxis medication, dosage, or length of prophylaxis. However, the task force agreed that some plastic surgery procedures warranted additional prophylaxis considerations; and accepted the premise that the surgical cases included in the orthopedic and general surgery literature search were similar enough in their anatomic location, degree of invasiveness and patient population to make them comparable (from a VTE risk perspective) to the following plastic surgery cases: major body contouring; abdominoplasty; major breast reconstruction; major lower extremity procedures; and major head/neck cancer procedure."[8] (VTE indicates venous thromboembolism.) Although there have been no randomized, controlled trials of chemoprophylaxis specific to plastic and reconstructive surgery, the validity of that approach was supported by the February 2012 publication of *Antithrombotic Therapy and Prevention of Thrombosis, 9th edition: American College of Chest Physicians Evidence-based Clinical Practice Guidelines*.[10]

Although some clinical practice guidelines regarding risk stratification and prevention were recommended in that referenced report, no definitive standard of care was established. At this time, the most definitive reviews of the literature and most clinically applicable guidelines for DVT prophylaxis are found in publications from the ASPS[8] and American Society for Aesthetic Plastic Surgery.[7]

Regardless of the risk stratification or algorithm used, if chemoprophylaxis is selected as part of the regimen, a full understanding of the basics of thrombus formation, of the available agents and how and why they work, as well as their associated risks, benefits and alternatives, is critical to their safest and most effective use. That is the focus of this article.

COAGULATION CASCADE

To understand the differences between the alternative chemoprophylaxis agents and how and why they work, at least a basic understanding of the coagulation cascade is necessary. The coagulation cascade is a series of enzymatic reactions that turns inactive precursors into active factors, the end result of which is the production of fibrin (factor I_a [FI_a]), a protein that serves as a glue to bind platelets and other materials together in a stable clot. The cascade has 2 initially separate, but then converging, pathways: the extrinsic pathway (which initiates coagulation in response to tissue injury, such as trauma or surgery) and the intrinsic pathway (so named because all the elements required for blood clotting are present, even in the absence of injury).

These two pathways converge to become a common pathway with the activation of factor X (FX) (**Fig. 1**). Active factors are indicated by the subscript a, whereas inactive precursors have no subscript.

THROMBUS FORMATION

The extrinsic pathway is initiated when tissue factor (TF), a transmembrane glycoprotein receptor in the subendothelial layers of blood vessels, is exposed to flowing blood following injury to the vessel. TF is rapidly bound by circulating factor VII (FVII). Binding is accompanied by autoactivation to FVII to form factor VII_a ($FVII_a$). The complex of TF and $FVII_a$ converts factor X (FX) into its active form, factor X_a (FX_a). FX_a subsequently binds factor V (FV) to form prothrombinase, the enzyme responsible for converting prothrombin into thrombin. In turn, thrombin converts fibrinogen to fibrin, initiating the clot.

In the intrinsic pathway, factor XI (FXI), which is found on activated platelets, is autoactivated to factor XI_a (FXI_a), which is capable of converting factor IX (FIX) to factor IX_a (FIX_a). (Again, the subscript a denotes the active form of a factor.) In turn, FIX_a activates FX in the presence of factor VIII (FVIII). At that point, the extrinsic and intrinsic pathways merge, with both causing the binding of FX_a to FV to form prothrombinase, the subsequent conversion of prothrombin into thrombin, and the thrombin-mediated formation of fibrin from fibrinogen. The extrinsic pathway can feed back into the intrinsic pathway as a result of thrombin-mediated activation of FXI, thus providing additional clotting support to seal a vascular injury.

Intrinsic control of the coagulation cascade and all of its interactions is necessary to maintain hemostatic balance. The extrinsic control and manipulation of that cascade is the focus in chemoprophylaxis of DVT. However, there is a difference between arterial and venous thrombus formation. Arterial thrombi consist primarily of platelet aggregates held together by small amounts of fibrin.[11] Because of that, strategies to inhibit arterial thrombogenesis focus primarily on drugs to disrupt platelet function. Venous thrombi are composed predominantly of fibrin and trapped

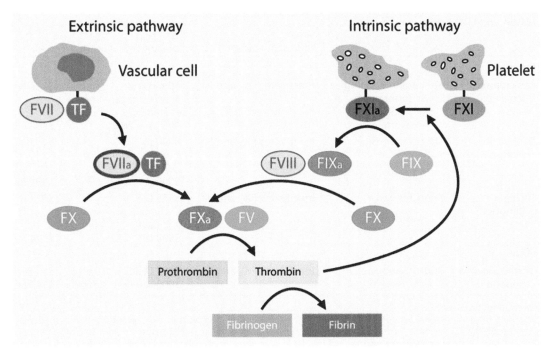

Fig. 1. A simplified overview of the coagulation cascade. TF, tissue factor. (*From* Colman RW. Are hemostasis and thrombosis two sides of the same coin? J Exp Med 2006;203:493–5; with permission.)

red blood cells with few platelets.[11] As a result, fibrinolytic agents are the focus for the treatment of venous thrombi. Although the development of new fibrinolytic agents has lagged behind that of antiplatelet and anticoagulant drugs,[10] there are still many agents from which clinicians can currently choose for DVT chemoprophylaxis, and many others under development.[12–14]

AGENTS FOR DVT CHEMOPROPHYLAXIS

Perhaps the easiest way to understand the approved and available anticoagulants useful for DVT chemoprophylaxis is to divide them into categories based on their mode of action, or their targets in the clotting cascade. For simplicity, this article divides them into heparins and nonheparins.

HEPARIN

Heparin, either low-molecular-weight heparin (LMWH) or low-density unfractionated heparin (LDUH), is perhaps the most widely used agent for DVT chemoprophylaxis. Both work through the same mechanism: the inactivation of FX_a and thrombin (FII_a) in the coagulation cascade.

One notable drawback to the heparins is that they also bind to cells and plasma proteins other than antithrombin, sometimes causing unpredictable pharmacokinetic and pharmacodynamic properties and triggering nonhemorrhagic side effects, such as heparin-induced thrombocytopenia (HIT) and, with long-term usage, osteoporosis.

However, LMWH has a significant advantage compared with LDUH in that it has greater inhibitory activity against FX_a than thrombin, and importantly binds less with plasma proteins, therefore having greater bioavailability.[7] The greater bioavailability of LMWH means that it can be given less frequently (once daily) because it has a longer plasma half-life, lower doses are usually required, it has a more predictable dose response, and therefore, unlike LDUH, it does not require constant coagulation monitoring. Based on those differences and their greater convenience, LMWHs have replaced unfractionated heparin for many clinical indications, including DVT prophylaxis. In addition, and importantly, although both LDUH and LMWH significantly reduce the rates of Symptomatic VTE, LMWH has been shown to be significantly more effective in reducing asymptomatic DVTs.[3]

NONHEPARINS

Unlike the heparins that specifically target FX_a and FII_a (thrombin), both the various currently available and investigational nonheparin anticoagulants applicable for DVT chemoprophylaxis target FII_a, $TF/FVII_a$, $FV_a/FVIII_a$, or FX_a directly or indirectly.

LMWA and LDUH drug comparison				
Drug	**Route**	**Mode of Action**	**Dosage and Duration**	**Cost**
LMWH				
Enoxaparin (Lovenox)	Subcutaneous (single-use syringes permitting self-injection)	Inactivates FX_a and FII_a	40 mg × 8 1 after surgery and 7 daily 40 mg × 28 d	$223.68 $782.88
Dalteparin (Fragmin)	Subcutaneous	Inactivates FX_a and FII_a	5000 IE × 8 1 after surgery and 7 daily 5000 IE × 28 d	$189.12 $661.92
Tinzaparin (Innohep)	Subcutaneous	Inactivates FX_a and FII_a	3500 IE × 8 1 after surgery and 7 daily 3500 IE × 28 d	$77.54 $274.40
LDUH				
Unfractionated heparin	Subcutaneous	Inactivates FX_a and FII_a	5000 U BID × 8 doses 5000 U BID × 8 doses	$40.80 $142.80

Abbreviation: BID, twice daily.

Modified from Murphy RX, Schmitz D, Rosolowski K, et al. Evidence-based practices for thromboembolism prevention: a report from the ASPS venous thromboembolism task force approved by the ASPS executive committee for publication. 2011. Available at: www.plasticsurgery.org.

Although there are numerous new subcutaneous antithrombotic drugs being investigated that work by a variety of mechanisms,[12] a similar comparison of the route of administration, dosage regimen, and cost of just the currently available nonheparin alternatives for DVT chemoprophylaxis is instructional (**Table 1**).

HEPARINS VERSUS NONHEPARINS

As with any other medications, there are risks and benefits to these alternatives. Although the LDUH risk of HIT or osteoporosis is significantly reduced with LMWH, because fondaparinux binds only to antithrombin, it essentially eliminates that risk. Both LMWH and fondaparinux exhibit significant bioavailability when administered subcutaneously, but fondaparinux has a longer half-life than LMWH. Both can be given once daily by subcutaneous injection in fixed doses, and neither requires coagulation monitoring. Although those are important considerations, two even more significant considerations are their relative effectiveness in preventing DVT and the risk of major bleeding.

Clinical trials indicate that fondaparinux is significantly more effective than LMWH (enoxoparin) in preventing postoperative DVT in joint replacement and hip fracture surgery. However, the

Table 1 Nonheparin antithrombotic drugs for DVT chemoprophylaxis				
Drug	**Route**	**Mode of Action**	**Dosage and Duration**	**Cost**
Fondaparinux (Arixtra)	Subcutaneous (single-use syringes permitting self-injection)	Indirectly inhibits FX_a Binds only to antithrombin	2.5 mg × 8 d 1 after surgery and 7 daily 2.5 mg × 28 d	$238.80 $825.80
Rivaroxaban (Xarelto)	Oral	Directly inhibits FX_a	10 mg PO QD	$280.00[a]
Dabigatran etexilate (Pradaxa)	Oral	Directly inhibits FII_a	75–150 mg PO BID	$140.00[a]

Abbreviations: BID, twice daily; PO, by mouth; QD, every day.
[a] For ease of comparison, this is based on average cost for an empiric 28 days of oral therapy.

From Murphy RX Jr, Alderman A, Gutowski K, et al. Evidence-based practices for thromboembolism prevention: summary of the ASPS Venous Thromboembolism Task Force Report. Plast Reconstr Surg 2012;130(1):168e–75e; with permission.

applicability of that finding to plastic surgery procedures is not definitive, and the results in multiple studies are mixed. Although some studies suggest that fondaparinux may cause more bleeding than LMWH, the incidence of clinically relevant bleeding was similar to that of LMWH, with the timing of the first dose of fondaparinux making the difference.[7] When the first dose of fondaparinux is given within 6 hours after surgery, more bleeding occurs than with enoxaparin. However, when the first dose is administered between 6 and 8 hours after surgery, bleeding rates are comparable. However, although bleeding problems after LMWH may be mitigated with the administration of protamine sulfate, if bleeding complications were to occur after fondaparinux there is no specific agent to reverse its anticoagulant effect. The patient would just have to be supported until the anticoagulant effects dissipate. The timing of administration also made a difference in DVT prevention, with fondaparinux being more effective in DVT prevention when given at least 6 hours after surgery than when given less than 6 hours after surgery (4.2% vs 6.5%, respectively).[7]

DVT CHEMOPROPHYLAXIS...OR NOT?

Despite the well-documented prevalence of DVT in surgical patients and the multiple risk assessment models proposing graded protocols for the use of DVT chemoprophylaxis, many plastic surgeons remain reluctant to use antithrombotic agents. However, most elective surgical patients do not have the common contraindications for anticoagulation, such as active bleeding, uncontrolled hypertension, HIT, coagulopathy, significant renal insufficiency, recent intraocular or intracranial surgery, or recent spinal tap. However, some surgeries may be done with epidural or spinal block, and many plastic surgeries involve the mobilization of large flaps of tissue and the creation of significant areas of dead space. The maintenance of meticulous hemostasis is critical to the success of plastic surgeries, and clinicians are wary of the risk of major bleeding, which can jeopardize our results. This caution does not mean that the bleeding has to be life threatening to cause significant problems in terms of flap or graft loss, wound disruption, scarring, hospitalization, prolonged recovery, and a suboptimal outcome. It is also difficult to accept the increased risk of even minor bleeding, which can cause limited hematoma and more extensive ecchymosis and edema and prolonged patient downtime. However, the risk of bleeding can be significantly minimized if the correct dose and dosage regimen of anticoagulation is used.

Table 2	
Recommended dosage and timing for DVT chemoprophylaxis agents	
Drug	**Dosage and Timing**
Enoxaparin (LMWH)	30–40 mg subcutaneously once daily. Initial dose 2 h before surgery or 12 h after surgery. Can continue until fully ambulatory, 5–10 d, or 7–12 d depending on estimated level of risk
Fondaparinux	2.5 mg subcutaneously once daily. Initial dose 6–8 h after surgery **(Never give before 6 h after surgery)**. Can continue for 7–12 d depending on estimated level of risk

Whatever risk assessment tools or protocol are followed, and whichever agent is selected for DVT chemoprophylaxis, the dosage and timing recommendations in **Table 2** should be appropriate.

SUMMARY

The practice of plastic surgery is a unique mixture of art and science, and both must be carefully balanced to provide the best possible care for patients. To do that, clinicians should ideally be practicing evidence-based medicine, which has been defined as "the conscientious, explicit and judicious use of current best evidence in making decisions about the care of individual patients."[15,16] It seeks to assess the strength of the evidence of the risks and benefits of treatments[17] to help clinicians predict whether a treatment will do more good than harm.[18] However, as noted earlier, the report from the ASPS Venous Thromboembolism Task Force concluded, as recently as July 2011, that "there was not enough evidence to make all-inclusive recommendations for plastic surgery prophylaxis medication, dosage, or length of prophylaxis."[8] This and the previous article emphasize the prevalence and risks associated with DVT and the reasons and options for its possible chemoprophylaxis. Until those evidence-based medicine best-practice recommendations can be developed, it would be prudent for clinicians to empirically select and consistently apply a risk stratification system and prophylaxis regimen of their choice for the benefit of their patients.

REFERENCES

1. US Department of Health and Human Services. The Surgeon General's call to action to prevent deep vein thrombosis and pulmonary embolism. 2008. Available at: http://www.surgeongeneral.gov/topics/deepvein/call toaction/call-to-action-on-dvt-2008.pdf.
2. Caprini JA. Thrombosis risk assessment as a guide to quality patient care. Dis Mon 2005;51:70–8.
3. Geerts WH, Pineo GF, Heit JA, et al. Prevention of venous thromboembolism: the Seventh ACCP Conference on Antithrombotic and Thrombolytic Therapy. Chest 2004;126(Suppl 3):338S–400S.
4. Bridges ND, Hellenbrand W, Latson L, et al. Transcatheter closure of patent foramen ovale after presumed paradoxical embolism. Circulation 1992;86(6):1902–8.
5. Messe SR, Silverman IE, Kizar JR, et al. Practice parameter: recurrent stroke with patent foramen ovale and atrial septal aneurysm: report of the Quality Standards Subcommittee of the American Academy of Neurology. Neurology 2004;62(7):1042–50.
6. Hirsh J, Bauer KA, Donati MB, et al. Parenteral anticoagulants: American College of Chest Physicians evidence-based clinical practice guidelines (8th edition). Chest 2008;133:141S–59S.
7. Young VL, Watson ME. The need for venous thromboembolism (VTE) prophylaxis in plastic surgery. Aesthet Surg J 2006;26(2):157–75.
8. Murphy RX, Schmitz D, Rosolowski K, et al. Evidence-based practices for thromboembolism prevention: a report from the ASPS Venous Thromboembolism Task Force approved by the ASPS Executive Committee for publication. 2011. Available at: www.plasticsurgery.org.
9. Heit JA, Rooke TW, Silverstein M, et al. Trends in the incidence of venous stasis syndrome and venous ulcer: a 25-year population-based study. J Vasc Surg 2001;33(5):1022–7.
10. Gould MK, Garcia DA, Wren SM, et al. Prevention of VTE in nonorthopedic surgical patients. Antithrombotic therapy and prevention of thrombosis, 9th edition: American College of Chest Physicians evidence-based clinical practice guidelines. Chest 2012;141(Suppl 2):e227S–77S.
11. Freiman D, Colman RW, Hirsh J, et al. The structure of thrombi, hemostasis and thrombosis: basic principles and clinical practice. 2nd edition. Philadelphia: JB Lippincott; 1987. p. 1123–35.
12. Weitz JI, Eikelboom JW, Samama MM. New antithrombotic drugs. Antithrombotic therapy and prevention of thrombosis, 9th edition: American College of Chest Physicians evidence-based clinical practice guidelines. Chest 2012;141(Suppl 2):e120S–51S.
13. Garcia DA, Baglin TP, Weitz JI, et al. Parenteral anticoagulants. Antithrombotic therapy and prevention of thrombosis, 9th edition: American College of Chest Physicians evidence-based clinical practice guidelines. Chest 2012;141(Suppl 2):e24S–43S.
14. Colman RW. Are hemostasis and thrombosis two sides of the same coin? J Exp Med 2006;203:493–5.
15. Sackett DL, Rosenberg WM, Gray JA, et al. Evidence based medicine; what it is and what it isn't. PubMed Central, Free Articles. BMJ 1996;312(7023):71–2.
16. Timmermans S, Mauck A. The promises and pitfalls of evidence-based medicine. Health Aff (Millwood) 2005;24(1):18–28.
17. Elstein AS. On the origins and development of evidence-based medicine and medical decision making. Inflamm Res 2004;53(Suppl 2):S184–9.
18. Atkins D, Best D, Briss PA, et al. Grading quality of evidence and strength of recommendations. BMJ 2004;328(7454):1490.

Airway Management in the Outpatient Setting

Katarzyna Luba, MD, MS*, Jeffrey L. Apfelbaum, MD,
Thomas W. Cutter, MD, MEd

KEYWORDS

- Airway management • Outpatient setting • Ambulatory surgery • Office-based surgery
- Outpatient surgery • Ambulatory anesthesia • Office-based anesthesia • Outpatient anesthesia

KEY POINTS

- Most cosmetic procedures are performed in outpatient surgical facilities with intravenous sedation, which may result in ventilatory depression and airway obstruction.
- Ventilatory and airway complications are a major factor in sedation-related adverse outcomes, such as death or anoxic brain injury.
- Appropriate patient and procedure selection may prevent ventilatory and airway-related complications.
- Preoperative patient evaluation may help identify patients at risk for airway complications but cannot rule out an unexpected difficult airway.
- All anesthetics should be administered by, or medically directed by, an anesthesiologist.
- The use of supplemental oxygen during sedation for procedures on the head, face, or neck creates a fire hazard.

INTRODUCTION

The type of airway management provided depends on the anesthetic technique and the type of anesthetic technique provided depends on the procedure. Although most outpatient cosmetic procedures are performed under minimal-to-moderate sedation with local anesthesia,[1] certain procedures require deep sedation or general anesthesia for patient comfort and cooperation. Occasionally, general anesthesia may be safer than deep sedation, especially in patients at risk for ventilatory or airway problems.

Sedation may be regarded as a continuum (**Table 1**) with the need for active airway management typically increasing as the depth of sedation increases.[2] Progression along this continuum is associated with diminished protective reflexes, including those that maintain ventilation, circulation, and airway patency and protection. Although the intention is to maintain one level of sedation, there is always the risk of progressing to the next level. Because of this risk, the anesthesia provider must be proficient in airway management commensurate with the level of sedation beyond that which is anticipated. The combination of a trained provider, appropriate patient and procedure selection, vigilance, and adherence to monitoring standards, can minimize anesthesia complications.

PREOPERATIVE PLANNING
Staff and Equipment

Administration of any level of sedation, ranging from moderate sedation through general anesthesia, requires a commensurate proficiency in

The authors have nothing to disclose.
Department of Anesthesia and Critical Care, University of Chicago, 5841 S. Maryland Avenue, MC 4028, Chicago, IL 60637, USA
* Corresponding author. Department of Anesthesia and Critical Care, The University of Chicago Medical Center, 5841 South Maryland Avenue, MC 4028, Chicago, IL 60637, USA.
E-mail address: kluba@dacc.uchicago.edu

Clin Plastic Surg 40 (2013) 405–417
http://dx.doi.org/10.1016/j.cps.2013.04.005

Table 1
Continuum of depth of sedation: definition of general anesthesia and levels of sedation and/or analgesia (Approved by ASA House of Delegates on October 13, 1999, and amended on October 27, 2004)

	Minimal Sedation (Anxiolysis)	Moderate Sedation and/or Analgesia (Conscious Sedation)	Deep Sedation and/or Analgesia	General Anesthesia
Responsiveness	Normal response to verbal stimulation	Purposeful* response to verbal or tactile stimulation	Purposeful* response following repeated or painful stimulation	Unarousable even with painful stimulus
Airway	Unaffected	No intervention required	Intervention may be required	Intervention often required
Spontaneous Ventilation	Unaffected	Adequate	May be inadequate	Frequently inadequate
Cardiovascular Function	Unaffected	Usually maintained	Usually maintained	May be impaired

* Reflex withdrawal from a painful stimulus is not considered a purposeful response.
Data from American Society of Anesthesiologists Task Force on Sedation and Analgesia by Non-Anesthesiologists. Practice guidelines for sedation and analgesia by non-anesthesiologists. Anesthesiology 2002;96(4):1004–17.

airway management and the equipment and supplies to execute it. The American Society of Anesthesiologists (ASA) guidelines for ambulatory anesthesia and office-based anesthesia[3,4] recommend that anesthesia beyond the level of moderate sedation be administered by anesthesiologists, or be medically directed by an anesthesiologist if administered by an anesthesia resident, a certified registered nurse anesthetist, or an anesthesia assistant. The ASA strongly recommends that, when an anesthesiologist is not available, non-physician anesthesia providers must be medically supervised by a licensed physician.[4] The medically supervising physician should be specifically trained in moderate or deep sedation[3] as well as airway, ventilation, and circulation rescue techniques (ie, management for one sedation level beyond that which is intended).[3,4] Specific sedation training for medical supervision is critical in office-based practices where hospital-based emergency backup is not immediately available.

Patients receiving moderate sedation are usually able to maintain a patent airway without assistance. Although supplemental oxygen may not be necessary, it should be available. Airway equipment for moderate sedation includes an oxygen source, nasal cannulas, suction catheters, oral and nasopharyngeal airways, and a means to administer positive pressure ventilation, such as a mask and artificial manual breathing unit (AMBU) bag. Deep sedation increases the risk of ventilatory depression and airway compromise, so additional equipment

must be available, including laryngoscopes, an assortment of several sizes of endotracheal tubes (ETTs), laryngeal mask airways (LMAs), and emergency surgical airway kits. The postanesthesia care unit should be outfitted similarly, based on the level of sedation performed intraoperatively and the need for postoperative sedation and analgesia.

Monitors should include pulse oximetry, ventilation (capnography or capnometry, ventilatory rate monitor), noninvasive blood pressure, continuous ECG, and temperature. A defibrillator and an emergency cart fully stocked with resuscitation drugs and equipment should be readily available[1] and the recovery room should be staffed by qualified nurses or other trained personnel.[1,3,5] Policies and protocols should be in place to respond to emergencies and to expedite patient transfers to an acute care hospital for extended care.[3,5]

Preoperative Fasting

Any level of sedation beyond minimal creates the potential for airway instrumentation. Preoperative fasting requirements must be observed before elective surgical procedures, except those performed with minimal sedation or without sedation. The ASA recommendations for preoperative fasting are given in **Table 2**.[6]

History and Physical Examination

The use of sedation may lead to an airway emergency, particularly if risk factors for a difficult airway

Table 2
American Society of Anesthesiologists guidelines for preoperative fasting

Food Ingested	Minimum Fasting Time Before Anesthesia
Clear liquid	2 h
Human milk	4 h
Infant formula, nonhuman milk	6 h
Light meal (eg, clear liquid + toast or cereal)	6 h
Meat or fat-containing food	8 h

have not been recognized preoperatively. The patient history can elicit past problems with anesthesia including difficulties with airway management. The physical examination may help identify a combination of features predictive of both airway and ventilatory complications.[7] In outpatient settings, airway evaluation may identify patients with an obvious or probable difficult airway, the management of which may require above-average expertise and skills, advanced techniques, expert assistance, and special equipment.

Predicting a difficult airway is simple only in a patient with a history of a difficult intubation, or with an obvious anatomy that suggests a difficulty. In other cases, a difficult airway is detected by recognizing a combination of subtle physical risk factors during an airway-focused physical examination (**Box 1**).[7]

According to the Mallampati classification (modified by Samsoon and Young[8]) there are four grades of visualization of the posterior pharyngeal structures, with classes 3 and 4 associated with a difficult exposure of the larynx during direct laryngoscopy[9] or difficult mask ventilation (**Fig. 1**).[10,11] Full extension at the atlanto-occipital joint should be at least 35° (**Fig. 2**). Cervical range of motion may be limited by previous trauma, surgical procedures, scarring from burns or radiation therapy, or a degenerative disease of the spine. Thyromental

Box 1
Elements of the airway examination

Transoral view of the posterior pharynx (Mallampati classification)

Range of motion of the cervical spine

Thyromental distance

Range of mouth opening

Mandibular protrusion test

Neck anatomy

Presence of a beard

Dentition

distance, from the mentum of the mandible to the superior margin of the thyroid cartilage, should be at least 6 cm or three average fingerbreadths (**Fig. 3**). Mouth opening is the measure of the distance between upper and lower incisors (or gingivae) and should be at least three fingerbreadths (**Fig. 4**). The mandibular protrusion test is normal if lower incisors can be protruded anterior to the upper incisors. It is limited in patients with a receding mandible (micrognathia) and overbite or limited mobility of the temporomandibular joint (**Fig. 5**). Neck anatomy may be significant for masses and motion-limiting scars or contractures and a short and thick neck may be associated with obstructive sleep apnea (OSA). A full beard interferes with mask ventilation because it prevents a tight seal between the mask and the face, and is often associated with micrognathia. Dentition should be inspected for the presence of removable dentures and loose teeth. Features that may interfere with laryngoscopy and intubation, especially when combined with other risk factors for a difficult airway, include protruding upper incisors, large upper crowns, or an oversized upper bridge (see **Fig. 5**). Earlier chin implants and genioplasties may produce a false thyromental distance and underestimation of the difficulty of maintaining an airway.

The anatomic features described above have limited sensitivity in predicting a difficult airway.[7] Most anesthesiologists evaluate a combination of several features to decide on the likelihood of a successful mask ventilation and intubation. The frequently used combination of the Mallampati score, range of flexion and extension of the neck, mouth opening, and thyromental distance suggests that difficult intubation is unlikely if these criteria are normal.[9]

Difficult or impossible mask ventilation may be associated with the presence of limited mandibular protrusion, low thyromental distance, obesity, snoring, or the presence of a beard.[10,11] Among patients with three or more predictors, mask ventilation was difficult in 5%, or 20 times the incidence in patients with no predictors.[11] Because mask

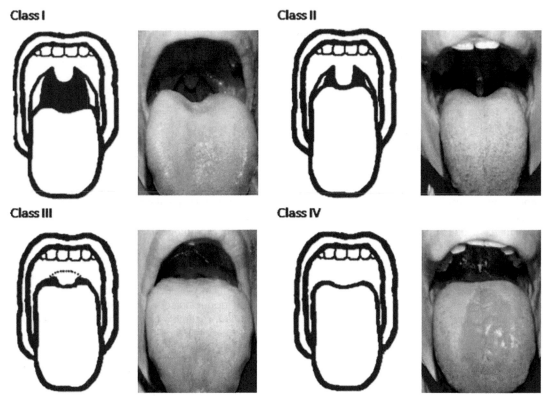

Fig. 1. Mallampati classification of oropharyngeal visualization modified by Samsoon and Young. (*From* Huang HH, Lee MS, Shih YL, et al. Modified Mallampati classification as a clinical predictor of peroral esophagogastroduodenoscopy tolerance. BMC Gastroenterol 2011;11:12.)

ventilation is the primary rescue technique for ventilatory depression or failed intubation, if difficult mask ventilation is anticipated, an anesthesiologist can formulate a backup plan for airway rescue before induction of general anesthesia or intravenous sedation. The criteria mentioned can help guide the selection of patients who may safely undergo procedures in a freestanding surgery center or a surgeon's office.

Morbidly obese patients are becoming more common, presenting airway and ventilatory management challenges. Obesity is a recognized risk

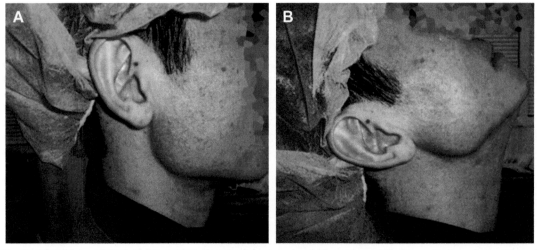

Fig. 2. (*A*) Neck in neutral position. (*B*) Full neck extension should be at least 35°. (*From* Orebaugh SL. Atlas of airway management: techniques and tools. Philadelphia: Lippincott Williams & Wilkins; 2007; with permission.)

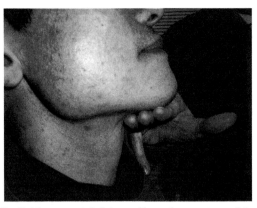

Fig. 3. Thyromental distance (from the mentum of the mandible to the upper margin of the thyroid cartilage) should be at least three average fingerbreadths. (*From* Orebaugh SL. Atlas of airway management: techniques and tools. Philadelphia: Lippincott Williams & Wilkins; 2007; with permission.)

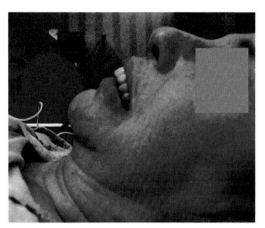

Fig. 5. Short mandible, overbite, and protruding incisor teeth. (*From* Orebaugh SL. Atlas of airway management: techniques and tools. Philadelphia: Lippincott Williams & Wilkins; 2007; with permission.)

factor for difficult mask ventilation.[10–12] However, difficult intubation is not more prevalent in the morbidly obese than in the general population[13–15] provided the patient has been placed in the ramped position for safe laryngoscopy and intubation (**Fig. 6**).[13] Pulmonary functional residual capacity is reduced in the morbidly obese;[12,16] therefore, the time to desaturation is much shorter than in normal-weight patients, especially in the supine position. A delay in securing the airway in an apneic, morbidly obese patient may rapidly lead to life-threatening hypoxemia. In the morbidly obese, a difficult airway correlates with male gender, Mallampati score of 3 or 4, and neck circumference greater than 40 cm.[14,15,17]

Obstructive sleep apnea (OSA) is a breathing disorder characterized by periodic upper airway obstruction during sleep.[18] Airway patency is restored by repetitive arousal from sleep, which may result in daytime hypersomnolence. OSA causes episodic hypoxemia and hypercarbia, which may lead to cardiovascular morbidity, including arrhythmias, systemic and pulmonary hypertension, and ischemic heart disease. The incidence of OSA is estimated at 1 in 4 in men and 1 in 10 in women in the general population,[18] but it is higher in the morbidly obese. There is a 70% incidence of OSA among patients undergoing bariatric surgery.[19]

OSA goes undiagnosed in approximately 80% to 90% of patients with the condition,[20] putting them at increased risk of anesthesia-related perioperative

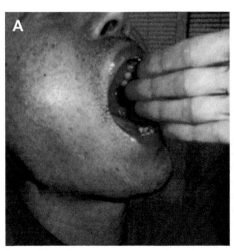
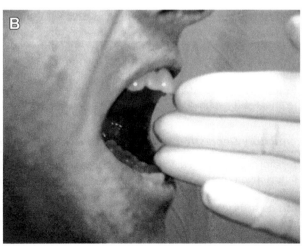

Fig. 4. (*A*) Full mouth opening should permit insertion of three fingers aligned vertically into the patient's mouth. (*B*) Limited mouth opening. (*From* Orebaugh SL. Atlas of airway management: techniques and tools. Philadelphia: Lippincott Williams & Wilkins; 2007; with permission.)

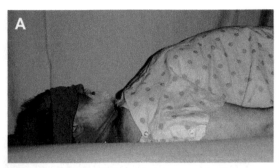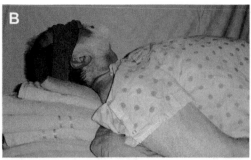

Fig. 6. (*A*) Morbidly obese patient in a standard supine position. This position creates misalignment of the laryngeal, pharyngeal and oral axis in the morbidly obese. (*B*) Morbidly obese patient in a ramped position for laryngoscopy and intubation. The external auditory meatus is aligned with the sternal notch, and the laryngeal, pharyngeal, and oral axis is aligned. (*Courtesy of* CR Enterprises, LLC, Frisco, TX; with permission.)

complications. Upper airway abnormalities that predispose to OSA also may result in difficult mask ventilation and intubation. Because patients with OSA are prone to airway obstruction during intravenous sedation, general anesthesia with a secured airway may be preferable to deep sedation. Another risk is ventilatory depression or arrest resulting from sedatives, opioids, and inhaled anesthetics.[18,21] This risk increases with postoperative administration of opioids for pain, and ventilatory depression is possible even on postoperative days 3 and 4 when sleep patterns are reestablished and "REM rebound" occurs.

Complications: Causes, Prevention, and Intraoperative Management

In the ASA Closed Claims database, the number of claims for anesthesia has decreased over the last three decades, but ventilatory complications remain a major cause, accounting for 17%, of all anesthesia claims between 1990 and 2007.[22] Ventilatory events that were most commonly associated with claims were difficult intubation, inadequate oxygenation or ventilation, and pulmonary aspiration. Permanent brain damage resulted in 8% to 10% of all anesthesia claims regardless of the anesthetic technique.[22]

Ventilatory Depression During Sedation

Propofol and opioids (eg, fentanyl, meperidine, sufentanil, hydromorphone, or morphine) are potent ventilatory depressants. Adding a benzodiazepine, such as midazolam, increases the risk of ventilatory depression. Oversedation with ventilatory depression accounted for 21% of claims with monitored anesthesia care (MAC).[22] Drug combinations (propofol with benzodiazepines or opioids) were involved in more than 50% of the cases.[22]

Risk factors for ventilatory depression during sedation with spontaneous ventilation include advanced age, OSA, and sleep deprivation. Because oxygen desaturation is a relatively late sign of ventilatory compromise, continuous monitoring of breathing by a dedicated provider is mandatory to recognize and treat ventilatory depression.[1] Observation of chest excursions, auscultation of breath sounds, and end-tidal capnography are useful for timely detection of ventilatory depression or airway obstruction.

Moderate ventilatory depression may respond to verbal and tactile stimulation and resolve after decreasing or discontinuing sedation, or after using airway maneuvers, such as chin lift or jaw thrust. If conservative measures are ineffective, the patient requires immediate bag-and-mask ventilation with supplemental oxygen. Mask ventilation may interfere with a surgical procedure, but supporting patient ventilation assumes priority. Placing an LMA or an ETT may ultimately be less disruptive than a mask. If the patient resumes breathing without an airway device, the subsequent decision to continue the procedure under a lighter level of sedation versus general anesthesia depends on the estimates of the risk of recurrence of ventilatory depression and the level of sedation required to continue the procedure.

Aspiration

Depression of protective airway reflexes with deep sedation or general anesthesia can lead to aspiration of stomach contents in patients with recent oral intake or delayed gastric emptying. This may result in atelectasis, pneumonitis, ventilatory failure, acute lung injury, or even death. Airway manipulation during LMA or ETT placement creates an additional aspiration risk, especially during repetitive attempts or emergency intubations. The

LMA is contraindicated for patients at risk for aspiration because it does not protect the airway.

To prevent aspiration, patients must be informed of preoperative fasting requirements, and compliance should be verified immediately before the procedure. In the event of noncompliance, the procedure should be canceled, postponed until the required fasting time elapses, or performed without sedation. In patients with chronic increased risk of aspiration (eg, gastroparesis or hiatal hernia), anesthesia choices include local or regional anesthesia with light sedation or without sedation, or general anesthesia with endotracheal intubation by a skilled provider. Deep sedation depresses protective airway reflexes and should be avoided. It also may create the need for rescue airway management, which is another risk factor for aspiration, particularly in a patient with a difficult airway. Pharmacologic agents, such as histamine-2 receptor agonists (ranitidine, famotidine) and proton pump inhibitors (omeprazole, lansoprazole) reduce gastric volume and acidity,[6] whereas metoclopramide reduces gastric volume.[6] Use of these agents may be helpful in patients at increased risk of aspiration in the immediate preoperative period.

Regurgitation and aspiration of a large volume of gastric contents is often obvious, but a silent aspiration during deep sedation or general anesthesia may go unnoticed. Aspiration during general anesthesia is more likely with an airway managed with an LMA, but even an ETT does not offer absolute protection against aspiration. The sequelae of aspiration may be immediate or delayed. Signs and symptoms are rales and rhonchi, wheezing (in about one-third of patients), increased inspiratory pressure during positive pressure ventilation, and hypoxemia. Patients who are awake may cough or show signs of stridor or ventilatory distress. Initial chest radiograph is often normal, but a massive or solid aspirate may result in immediate atelectasis, commonly of the right lower lobe.

To manage aspiration, the upper airway should be suctioned to clear obstructive material. If necessary, ventilation and oxygenation via endotracheal intubation may be used, allowing for suctioning of the trachea and bronchi. A fiberoptic bronchoscope may be helpful in identifying and removing any large chunks of aspirated material. Irrigating the lower airways is not useful, and prophylactic antibiotics and corticosteroids are not indicated.[23]

Laryngospasm

Laryngospasm is a reflex spasm of the striated muscles of the larynx, resulting in partial or complete closure of the glottis and an inability to ventilate the lungs. Laryngospasm has the potential to cause serious complications, including death. A patient under sedation or general anesthesia whose airway is not protected by an ETT may experience laryngospasm, or it may be precipitated by airway manipulation (extubation, insertion of an LMA or an oropharyngeal tube, or suctioning), by blood or secretions in the pharynx, vomiting, patient movement, surgical stimulus during light anesthesia, or an irritant volatile anesthetic. Signs include inspiratory stridor, complete airway obstruction, increased inspiratory efforts, paradoxic chest and abdominal movements, suprasternal tug, desaturation, and bradycardia.

Airway patency may be restored with jaw thrust and positive pressure mask ventilation with 100% oxygen. Deepening anesthesia with a rapidly acting intravenous agent, such as propofol, is frequently beneficial. If these measures fail, a muscle relaxant, typically succinylcholine, is administered. Succinylcholine is short-acting, so endotracheal intubation may not be necessary. Mask ventilation until the return of spontaneous breathing is often sufficient. The patient may be intubated in the event of difficult mask ventilation or other problems. The complications of laryngospasm include aspiration and negative inspiratory pressure pulmonary edema, and the patient may require ventilatory support in an intensive care setting.[24]

Airway Obstruction

The airway may be obstructed during moderate or deep sedation. Risk factors include OSA, obesity, a receding mandible, and neurologic disorders with pharyngeal muscle weakness (eg, cerebral palsy, amyotrophic lateral sclerosis).

Airway obstruction must be recognized as soon as it occurs. Monitoring end-tidal expiratory carbon dioxide (CO_2) and pulse oximetry is the standard of care for all patients given moderate sedation and is mandatory during deep sedation. If monitoring end-tidal CO_2 is not feasible during moderate sedation, airway obstruction may be recognized by lack of breath sounds on chest auscultation. Paradoxic chest wall and diaphragm movements in a patient with an obstructed airway may be mistaken for normal chest excursions, so it is crucial to confirm effective air movement or perform maneuvers to restore airway patency. A decline in oxygen saturation is a late finding and never the first indication of an obstruction.

If an airway is obstructed, both sedation and the surgical procedure should be discontinued. Persistent airway obstruction inevitably leads to desaturation. In a morbidly obese patient, profound hypoxemia will follow rapidly. Dentures should be removed and effective maneuvers to open an obstructed upper airway instituted, including tilting the head back or turning it sideways, lifting the chin, thrusting the jaw forward, and placing an oropharyngeal or nasopharyngeal airway.[25] These maneuvers may be combined with positive pressure mask ventilation. If unsuccessful, an LMA or an ETT should be placed.

Hypoxemia that persists after ventilation is restored with 100% oxygen raises a suspicion of aspiration or postobstructive negative inspiratory pressure pulmonary edema. These conditions may require intubation, ventilation and transfer to a critical care setting.[25]

Airway Crisis: "Cannot Ventilate, Cannot Intubate"

Adverse outcomes have declined since the adoption of the ASA practice guidelines for management of the difficult airway.[7] However, because of the consequences of the "cannot ventilate, cannot intubate" scenario, the importance of preoperative airway evaluation to identify patients with a difficult airway cannot be overemphasized. The strategy for the management of a known difficult airway includes having a trained anesthesia provider, an expert assistant, and specialized difficult airway equipment stored in a readily accessible, portable unit (**Box 2**).[7]

Persistent intubation attempts during an airway crisis have been associated with death or permanent brain damage,[22] so they should be limited to three before attempting placement of an LMA.[22] If ventilation with an LMA is unsuccessful at first attempt, a surgical airway should be promptly secured (**Fig. 7**)[22]; therefore, the surgeon or anesthesiologist must be trained in emergency invasive airway access, such as tracheostomy or cricothyroidotomy. Difficult airway management, even in an elective scenario, may result in aspiration or airway trauma and the patient may remain intubated for airway protection and ventilatory support. In the event of complications, a ventilator and nursing staff familiar with the care of a patient whose lungs are mechanically ventilated must be available and the facility must have a policy and a protocol for patient transfer to an acute care hospital.[3,5] Unless all these requirements are met, a patient with a known or suspected difficult airway should not have a procedure in an outpatient facility. The single exception is for a surgical procedure performed with minimal sedation.

Operating Room Fire

On-the-patient operating room (OR) fires account for nearly a fifth of MAC-related closed claims.[22] Almost all of these events occurred during surgery on the head, face, or neck in the presence of

---

Box 2
Contents of the portable storage unit for management of a difficult airway[a]

1. Rigid laryngoscope blade of alternate design and size from those routinely used; this may include a rigid fiberoptic laryngoscope

2. Tracheal tubes of assorted sizes

3. Tracheal tube guides. Examples include, but are not limited to, semirigid stylets, ventilating tube changer, light wands, and forceps to manipulate the distal portion of the tracheal tube.

4. LMAs of assorted sizes; this may include the intubating LMA and the LMA ProSeal (LMA North America, Inc, San Diego, CA, USA)

5. Flexible fiberoptic intubation equipment

6. Retrograde intubation equipment

7. At least one device suitable for emergency noninvasive airway ventilation. Examples include, but are not limited to, an esophageal tracheal Combitube (Kendall-Sheridan Catheter Corp, Argyle, NY, USA), a hollow jet ventilation stylet, and a transtracheal jet ventilator

8. Equipment suitable for emergency invasive airway access (eg, cricothyroidotomy)

9. An exhaled CO_2 detector

[a] The items listed are suggestions. The contents of the portable storage unit should be customized to meet the specific needs, preferences, and skills of the practitioner and health care facility.
Adapted from American Society of Anesthesiologists (ASA) Task Force on Management of the Difficult Airway. Practice guidelines for management of the difficult airway. An updated report by the American Society of Anesthesiologists Task Force on Management of the Difficult Airway. Anesthesiology 2003;98:1269–77; with permission.

---

electrocautery and supplemental oxygen.[26] OR fires may cause burns, inhalation injury, infection, disfigurement, or even death.

An OR fire requires the presence of the fire triad: ignition source (cautery or laser), oxidizer (supplemental oxygen), and fuel (drapes, sponges, airway devices, and alcohol-based prepping solutions).[26] Surgery on the face, head, or neck brings the ignition source (cautery or laser) near an oxygen-enriched atmosphere, creating a high risk of fire. OR fires may be prevented by collaboration and communication between the surgical, nursing, and anesthesia teams before and during the procedure. If light sedation is sufficient, supplemental oxygen may be omitted. Otherwise, the fraction of

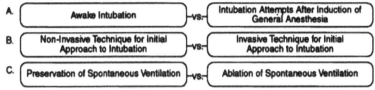

DIFFICULT AIRWAY ALGORITHM

1. Assess the likelihood and clinical impact of basic management problems:
    A. Difficult Ventilation
    B. Difficult Intubation
    C. Difficulty with Patient Cooperation or Consent
    D. Difficult Tracheostomy

2. Actively pursue opportunities to deliver supplemental oxygen throughout the process of difficult airway management

3. Consider the relative merits and feasibility of basic management choices:

    A. Awake Intubation —vs.— Intubation Attempts After Induction of General Anesthesia

    B. Non-Invasive Technique for Initial Approach to Intubation —vs.— Invasive Technique for Initial Approach to Intubation

    C. Preservation of Spontaneous Ventilation —vs.— Ablation of Spontaneous Ventilation

4. Develop primary and alternative strategies:

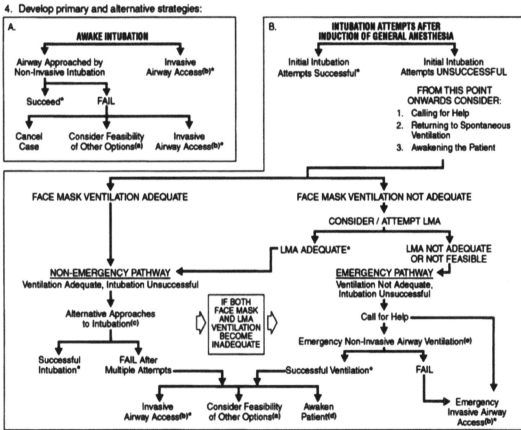

* Confirm ventilation, tracheal intubation, or LMA placement with exhaled CO_2

a. Other options include (but are not limited to): surgery utilizing face mask or LMA anesthesia, local anesthesia infiltration or regional nerve blockade. Pursuit of these options usually implies that mask ventilation will not be problematic. Therefore, these options may be of limited value if this step in the algorithm has been reached via the Emergency Pathway.

b. Invasive airway access includes surgical or percutaneous tracheostomy or cricothyrotomy.

c. Alternative non-invasive approaches to difficult intubation include (but are not limited to): use of different laryngoscope blades, LMA as an intubation conduit (with or without fiberoptic guidance), fiberoptic intubation, intubating stylet or tube changer, light wand, retrograde intubation, and blind oral or nasal intubation.

d. Consider re-preparation of the patient for awake intubation or canceling surgery.

e. Options for emergency non-invasive airway ventilation include (but are not limited to): rigid bronchoscope, esophageal-tracheal combitube ventilation, or transtracheal jet ventilation.

Fig. 7. An algorithm for management of a difficult airway. (*From* American Society of Anesthesiologists (ASA) Task Force on Management of the Difficult Airway. Practice guidelines for management of the difficult airway. An updated report by the American Society of Anesthesiologists Task Force on Management of the Difficult Airway. Anesthesiology 2003;98:1269–77; with permission.)

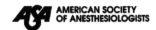
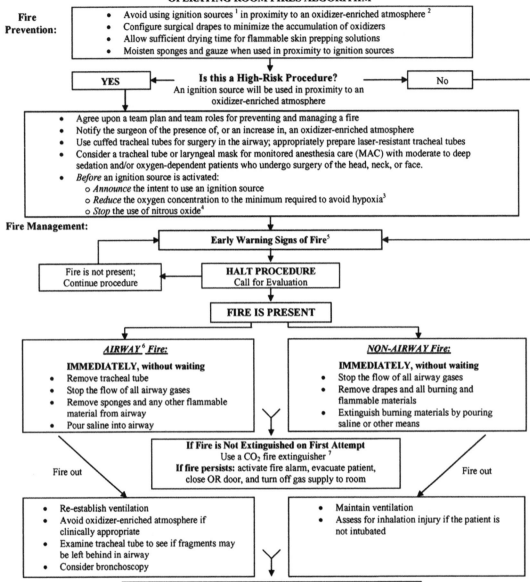

Fig. 8. An algorithm for preventing fires in the OR. (*From* American Society of Anesthesiologists (ASA) Task Force on Operating Room Fires. Practice advisory for the prevention and management of operating room fires. Anesthesiology 2008;108:786–801; with permission.)

inspired oxygen (F$_{IO_2}$) should be kept to a minimum in the proximity of electrocautery, or a sealed inspiratory gas delivery with an ETT or LMA should be considered. If an open oxygen delivery system (facemask or nasal cannula) is used, several precautions should be taken. Flammable skin prepping solutions must be allowed to dry before draping, surgical drapes should be open to the room to minimize the accumulation of oxygen under the drapes, the operating field should be scavenged with suction, and gauze and sponges in the proximity of the cautery should be moistened. Finally, the surgeon should give the anesthesiologist adequate notice before using cautery or a laser beam so he or she may discontinue or minimize the delivery of oxygen and then wait for several minutes for it to dissipate. The patient should be monitored with pulse oximetry for tolerance of decreased oxygen.

In the event of a fire, the procedure is stopped immediately, burning and flammable materials are removed from the patient, oxygen delivery is discontinued, and the airway is evaluated and secured. The patient is assessed for smoke inhalation injury (**Fig. 8**).[26]

Postoperative Management

Most patients who have experienced perioperative airway-related complications require extended observation in the recovery room. In cases of severe complications, postoperative care involves active management of the sequelae while arrangements are made to transfer the patient to a hospital. Recovery room personnel should be qualified to monitor ventilatory function, to respond to and assist with airway emergencies, and to care for an intubated patient.

Patients who experience ventilatory depression or partial airway obstruction under sedation and who have no other risk factors may be discharged from the outpatient facility after observation in the recovery room. Patients who had a severe airway obstruction or laryngospasm will probably need postoperative assessment to rule out aspiration and pulmonary edema. The patient is observed for initiation or worsening of ventilatory distress or hypoxemia.

Airway complications that may necessitate transfer to an acute care facility include bronchospasm, unexpected difficult airway, traumatic intubation, and on-the-patient OR fire, regardless of the need to keep the patient intubated in the postoperative period. These complications have the potential to evolve into delayed ventilatory distress, ventilatory failure, or airway compromise, even if the patient's condition initially seems stable. In the case of a witnessed aspiration or an emergent difficult airway, the patient should remain intubated and receive ventilatory support, sedation, and airway care in the outpatient facility until transfer to a hospital.

Postoperative hypoxemia often develops from ventilatory depression, atelectasis, airway obstruction, pulmonary edema, or aspiration. Supplemental oxygen is administered to all obese or OSA patients during the recovery phase and they should be considered for discharge only when oxygen saturation on room air returns to their preoperative baseline.

Ventilatory depression may result from residual perioperative sedation or opioid analgesics. Intravenous opioid and benzodiazepine antagonists (naloxone and flumazenil) should be available to reverse ventilatory depression.[1] The duration of action of these antagonists is often shorter than that of the drugs they reverse and ventilatory depression may recur; therefore, continued observation and monitoring is mandatory.

Postoperative airway obstruction is life threatening and may result from residual sedation, residual neuromuscular blockade, or airway trauma. Symptoms of airway trauma may include hoarseness, dysphonia, cough, stridor, pain, suprasternal tug, and ventilatory distress. Airway obstruction from residual sedation or neuromuscular blockade may be managed initially by bag and mask ventilation, but worsening of symptoms should hasten the decision to intubate the patient.

Patients with OSA are a particular concern in the outpatient setting because of the high risk of postoperative ventilatory depression and airway obstruction.[18,21,27] Anesthetic choices in these patients minimize the use of sedatives and opioids. Patients with severe OSA are considered questionable candidates for outpatient procedures with sedatives or opioids.[18,27] Patients who use continuous positive airway pressure should have it available during recovery. Before discharge from the facility, patients with OSA should be monitored for up to 3 hours longer than non-OSA patients.[18] If they develop an episode of airway obstruction or desaturation during sleep while breathing room air in an unstimulated environment, monitoring should continue for another 7 hours before discharge from the facility.[18]

SUMMARY

The past few decades have seen a significant and widely recognized improvement in the safety of anesthesia. However, complications related to airway management remain a major factor in anesthesia-related poor outcomes, such as anoxic brain injury and death.

Most outpatient cosmetic procedures are now performed in surgeons' offices, with patients under local anesthesia and minimal intravenous sedation. Sedation at any level beyond minimal creates the risk of airway obstruction and ventilatory depression, which can result in irreversible brain injury or death within minutes. The outcome of an airway management issue critically depends on the skills and expertise of the providers, and on the availability of appropriate specialized equipment. Because outpatient surgical facilities may lack the requisite expertise and equipment, preoperative patient evaluation should help identify and exclude patients at risk for airway complications. One must also be prepared for the unexpected difficult airway and, to minimize the risk of an adverse outcome of an airway-related complication, all anesthetics should be administered or medically directed by an anesthesiologist. If an anesthesiologist is unavailable, a non-physician anesthesia provider should be medically supervised by a licensed physician trained in airway rescue techniques.

OSA, a relatively common and often undiagnosed condition, places patients at an increased risk for ventilatory depression, and such patients are often poor candidates for outpatient procedures with the use of opioids and sedatives. In addition, many cosmetic procedures performed with intravenous sedation create an increased risk of an OR fire by bringing together the fire triad (electrocautery or lasers, supplemental oxygen, and flammable materials). Careful preoperative planning and effective intraoperative communication among all members of the OR team are necessary to avoid this and other airway complications.

REFERENCES

1. Bitar G, Mullis W, Jacobs W, et al. Safety and efficacy of office-based surgery with monitored anesthesia care/sedation in 4778 consecutive plastic surgery procedures. Plast Reconstr Surg 2003; 11:150–6.
2. American Society of Anesthesiologists. Practice guidelines for sedation and analgesia by non-anesthesiologists. Anesthesiology 2002;96:1004–17.
3. American Society of Anesthesiologists (ASA). Guidelines for ambulatory anesthesia and surgery. Available at: http://www.asahq.org/publications-Guidelines-for-Ambulatory-Anesthesia-and-Surgery. (Approved by the ASA House of Delegates on October 15, 2003, and last amended on October 21, 2008). Accessed October 10, 2012.
4. American Society of Anesthesiologists (ASA). Statement on qualifications of anesthesia providers in the office-based setting. Available at: http://www.asahq. org/publications-statement-on-Qualifications-of-Anesthesia-Providers-in-the-Office-Based-Setting. (Approved by the ASA House of Delegates on October 13, 1999, and last amended October 21, 2009). Accessed October 10, 2012.
5. American Society of Anesthesiologists (ASA). Guidelines for office-based anesthesia. Available at: http://www.asahq.org/publications-guidelines-for-Office-Based-Anesthesia.pdf. (Approved by the ASA House of Delegates on October 13, 1999, and last affirmed on October 21, 2009). Accessed October 10, 2012.
6. American Society of Anesthesiologists (ASA) Committee on Standards and Practice Parameters. Practice guidelines for preoperative fasting and the use of pharmacologic agents to reduce the risk of pulmonary aspiration: application to healthy patients undergoing elective procedures. Anesthesiology 2011;114:495–511.
7. American Society of Anesthesiologists (ASA) Task Force on Management of the Difficult Airway. Practice guidelines for management of the difficult airway. An updated report by the American Society of Anesthesiologists Task Force on Management of the Difficult Airway. Anesthesiology 2003;98:1269–77.
8. Samsoon GL, Young JR. Difficult tracheal intubation: a retrospective study. Anaesthesia 1987;42:487–90.
9. Orebaugh SL. Definitions, incidence and predictors of the difficult airway. In: Orebaugh SL, editor. Atlas of airway management: techniques and tools. Philadelphia: Lippincott Williams & Wilkins; 2007. p. 39–47.
10. Langeron O, Masso E, Huraux C, et al. Prediction of difficult mask ventilation. Anesthesiology 2000;92: 1229–36.
11. Kheterpal S, Han R, Tremper KK, et al. Incidence and predictors of difficult and impossible mask ventilation. Anesthesiology 2006;105:885–91.
12. Adams JP, Murphy PG. Obesity in anaesthesia and intensive care. Br J Anaesth 2000;85:91–108.
13. Nelligan PJ. Metabolic syndrome: anesthesia for morbid obesity. Curr Opin Anaesthesiol 2010;23: 375–83.
14. Nelligan PJ, Porter S, Max B, et al. Obstructive sleep apnea is not a risk factor for difficult intubation in morbidly obese patients. Anesth Analg 2009;109: 1182–6.
15. Ezri T, Medalion B, Weisenberg M, et al. Increased body mass index per se is not a predictor of difficult laryngoscopy. Can J Anaesth 2003;50:179–83.
16. Biring MS, Lewis MI, Liu JT, et al. Pulmonary physiologic changes of morbid obesity. Am J Med Sci 1999;318:293–7.
17. Brodsky JB, Lemmens HJ, Brock-Utne JG, et al. Morbid obesity and tracheal intubation. Anesth Analg 2002;94:732–6.
18. Gross JB, Bachenberg KL, Benumof JL, et al. American Society of Anesthesiologists (ASA) Task

Force on Perioperative Management of Patients with Obstructive Sleep Apnea. Practice guidelines for the perioperative management of patients with obstructive sleep apnea. Anesthesiology 2006;104:1081–93.

19. Frey WC, Pilcher J. Obstructive sleep-related breathing disorders in patients evaluated for bariatric surgery. Obes Surg 2003;13:676–83.

20. Hallowell PT, Stellato TA, Schuster M, et al. Potentially life-threatening sleep apnea is unrecognized without aggressive evaluation. Am J Surg 2007; 193:364–7.

21. Tung A. Anaesthetic considerations with the metabolic syndrome. Br J Anaesth 2010;105(Suppl 1):i24–33.

22. Metzner J, Posner KL, Lam MS, et al. Closed claims' analysis. Best Pract Res Clin Anaesthesiol 2011;25: 263–76.

23. Marik PE. Aspiration pneumonitis and aspiration pneumonia. N Engl J Med 2001;344:665–71.

24. Visvanathan T, Kluger MT, Webb RK, et al. Crisis management during anesthesia: laryngospasm. Qual Saf Health Care 2005;14:e3. Available at: http://www.qshc.com/cgi/content/full/14/3/e3. Accessed May 10, 2013.

25. Visvanathan T, Kluger MT, Webb RK, et al. Crisis management during anesthesia: obstruction of the natural airway. Qual Saf Health Care 2005;14:e2. Available at: http://www.qshc.com/cgi/content/full/14/3/e2. Accessed May 10, 2013.

26. American Society of Anesthesiologists (ASA) Task Force on Operating Room Fires. Practice advisory for the prevention and management of operating room fires. Anesthesiology 2008;108:786–801.

27. Ankichetty S, Chung F. Considerations for patients with obstructive sleep apnea undergoing ambulatory surgery. Curr Opin Anaesthesiol 2011;24: 605–11.

Endoscopy in the Outpatient Setting

Michael Frank, MD[a,b]

KEYWORDS

- Gastrointestinal endoscopy • Outpatients • Anesthesia • Complications

KEY POINTS

- Office endoscopy is an accepted safe alternative to in-hospital care. Attention to detail will help to ensure that the vast majority of procedures will be successfully completed without incident.
- An office setting offers advantages for the patient and the endoscopist.
- The office should be able to personalize the care and minimize what might be a stressful and anxiety-provoking visit.
- The physician will be able to work at his or her own pace with staff that knows exactly how each procedure will be performed. The physician should assure the patient that in this office every detail has been carefully scrutinized for the patient's care and safety.
- Recognizing a complication and taking all steps to rectify the situation in a timely and appropriate fashion is important for the patient's well-being.
- Patients' safety depends on a well-designed infrastructure and a staff that works together harmoniously in a facility that calls for constant support and attention to detail and not simply a skilled endoscopist.

Editorial Comment: Rationale for including gastrointestinal endoscopy in Plastic Surgery issue:

The author presents safe practice of endoscopy in the outpatient setting, focused primarily on gastrointestinal endoscopy. Why is this of interest to plastic surgeons? Principles for safe endoscopy apply to plastic surgery in the same way that they apply to gastrointestinal surgery. The plastic surgeon will be interested to read the recommendations for and pitfalls of endoscopy in the ambulatory setting that discuss anesthesia, complications, and more.

INTRODUCTION TO GENERAL ENDOSCOPY

- Endoscopy units have evolved over the past 50 years from small rooms usually placed at the far end of a general medical floor or single multipurpose units as part of the operating room to large, stand-alone suites either in or outside of a hospital, with multiple rooms to accommodate many diagnostic and advanced therapeutic procedures. Indications for endoscopy have also changed over time. Today diagnostic procedures are commonly performed on asymptomatic patients to identify premalignant conditions in those who are at high risk of developing cancer, and more commonly on healthy people for screening. Highly complex therapeutic procedures such as endomucosal resection and biliary interventions have become outpatient procedures performed in specialty units or even in private offices. The movement from a hospital setting to the outpatient facility is the result of multiple factors.
- Scheduling pressures for endoscopy time crowded many hospital endoscopy units so that endoscopists looked to perform procedures in an alternative location, leaving hospital suites available for in-patient care.
- Insurance reimbursement incentivized endoscopy performance outside of the hospital.

[a] New York University School of Medicine, 550 1st Avenue, New York, New York 10016, USA; [b] Lenox Hill Hospital, New York, New York, USA
E-mail address: mikefrankmd@gmail.com

Clin Plastic Surg 40 (2013) 419–427
http://dx.doi.org/10.1016/j.cps.2013.04.006
0094-1298/13/$ – see front matter © 2013 Elsevier Inc. All rights reserved.

- Physicians themselves found they had more control of their time and even the quality of the endoscopy if performed under their direct guidance and leadership rather than in the hospital.

Today, numerous sites of service are available for endoscopy including ambulatory endoscopy centers (AECs), ambulatory surgery centers (ASCs), or a physician's own private office.

In his review on safe endoscopy published in *Gastrointestinal Endoscopy* in 1994, the late Emmet Keeffe wrote, "Endoscopy is probably safer in a large hospital endoscopy unit than a small rural hospital procedure room, although this hypothesis has not been studied." Today, safe office endoscopy has come of age. What are the advantages of endoscopy in the office setting and why do most patients prefer to have their procedures outside of a hospital?

- Patients who are generally healthy prefer to remain out of the hospital.
- Patients are more comfortable seeing their physician in the facility where they may be familiar with the location, the personnel, and a routine they have grown accustomed to.
- Patients do not want to share a waiting room with sick inpatients in wheelchairs or on stretchers, or be inconvenienced by delays in the schedule forced on them by unforeseen emergencies.
- In hospital, patients are interviewed by multiple staff in a unit with many asking the same questions. Sometimes more than 1 to 2 hours have elapsed from entry point until the procedure begins.
- Patients are concerned about effects of anesthesia and possible complications, primarily infections and perforation.[1]

Why do physicians want to do procedures outside a hospital?

- A physician has better control over time management when working in his or her own office. The surgeon is able to examine a patient in between procedures, maximizing efficiency.
- Procedures can be scheduled in a sequence that conforms to an individual style and patient load.
- In a hospital setting, the endoscopist has limited flexibility because multiple physicians have to be accommodated and time must often be reserved for potential emergencies. Many hospitals host fellowship training programs whereby endoscopic teaching and learning may add extensive time to the

procedure. The result is that in-hospital endoscopy time estimates are often inaccurate and delays are normative.

Although there are regional differences, in many parts of North America office endoscopy has become mainstream, with the office a preferred location for common procedures. However, quality endoscopy is more complex than just clean scopes and clean rooms. The purpose of this article is to highlight many issues that serve to make office endoscopy a safe alternative to the hospital-based procedure.

STANDARDS FOR OFFICE ENDOSCOPY

The American Society of Gastrointestinal Endoscopy has stated that the standards for out-of-hospital endoscopic practice should be identical to the recognized guidelines followed in the hospital.[2] To achieve this goal many states have adopted mandatory accreditation from national organizations such as the Joint Commission on Accreditation of Health Care Organizations, the American Association of Ambulatory Surgery Facilities, and the Accreditation Association for Ambulatory Health Care. These organizations are dedicated to maintaining a high standard of care in the office setting. Even where those standards are not regulated by law, out-of-hospital endoscopy relies on the physicians' and staff's devotion to patient safety and comfort. Rules and forms are important, but an office and its entire staff should strive to establish a goal of excellence, with all personnel made to understand the value and importance of a safe environment.

PERSONNEL

The office staff is usually a patient's first contact with an endoscopy center. The reliability and caliber of office personnel is second in importance to that of the physician's. The clarity, compassion, and concern expressed by the staff are a direct reflection of how important the physician values the safety and welfare of the patient. The office personnel and the clinical staff must be able work together to promote a congenial environment with a common goal dedicated to the well-being of the patients served.

The office staff is often the filter between patient and physician. In outpatient endoscopy units it is imperative that the staff understand the procedures performed by the physician. Staff must understand the importance of the preparation and be able to instruct the patients how to prepare for their procedure. The staff may be asked to triage patients and schedule their access to the physician, based on their specific medical problems. Staff must be trained and educated on the basic issues that patients may inquire about and be capable of referring a patient's telephone inquiry to either nurses or physicians. Failure to recognize a patient's problem as critical or life-threatening can delay and complicate the patient's care and access to the physician. For example, a complaint of pain or bleeding should be referred to a nurse or physician to determine the urgency of a visit or need for emergent care.

The staff needs to understand procedure scheduling to allow enough time between procedures for room preparation, equipment processing, and patient setup. Failure to allow appropriate time between procedures will make the physician feel rushed to complete the examination to minimize prolonged waiting time. Every effort should be made to keep waiting time for patients to a minimum. A well-run office will inform a patient if there is an anticipated delay. The patient must be treated with care and dignity by the staff at all times. An office that understands the value of the patient's time and appreciates their anxiety on the day of the procedure is one that will engender confidence that the technical aspects of the endoscopy will be handled with the utmost care. An office that is habitually running hours behind schedule with a waiting room filled with unhappy, irritated, and anxious patients, by contrast, will likely call into question the competency and reliability of the endoscopist.

Although the physician decides which medications need to be discontinued before the procedure (in collaboration with other treating physicians), the staff often communicates these instructions to the patient directly. Instructions about aspirin and other anticoagulation can often be confusing for a patient who is anxious about his or her upcoming procedure. Anecdotally, the author can recall a patient who came for a procedure and who had assured the interviewing nurses that he took neither coumadin nor aspirin. On observing a gush of blood from the base of the stalk after polypectomy, he explained that he took warfarin, but was not specifically asked about that product. Today there are many new antiplatelet agents and anticoagulants, and it is critical to record the medications taken by a prospective patient and advise on its use or discontinuation. The decision to discontinue anticoagulation is usually made after discussion with other treating physicians.

The endoscopy assistant is another key person whose experience and knowledge will enhance a safe environment. The assistant can be a registered nurse, a licensed practical nurse, or a trained technician. If the assistant is working alone with the endoscopist, he or she may assist in the performance of biopsy or polypectomy. In patients who require more intensive or prolonged endoscopic interventions, a second assistant would be needed to allow the assistant administering moderate sedation to remain focused on patient monitoring rather than technical assistance.[2] Even if the assistant is a nurse, his or her educational background or experience with anesthetized patients may be limited. Teaching and training until the assistant feels comfortable and confident with the responsibilities cannot be overstated. Training an assistant requires time and patience. No one should be thrown into the position and be expected to learn "on the job" while doing procedures. Training may be available at the local hospital, where a new employee might be able to observe the entire outpatient endoscopy routine over several weeks before joining the office endoscopy unit. The assistant's responsibilities must be clearly delineated. Responsibility may also include care for the equipment, which can be learned from the manufacturer's representative, who may have a clinical coordinator who will come into the office and provide direct instructions on care of the instruments.

PREPROCEDURE EVALUATION

Under ideal conditions a patient should undergo a complete medical history and physical and appropriate laboratory examination before any procedure. Routine tests including coagulation studies, chest radiograph, electrocardiogram, blood cross-matching, hemoglobin level, urinalysis, and chemistry tests are not recommended before endoscopy.[3] However, the indication for the procedure should be carefully explained as well as alternatives and risks involved with the planned procedure. Information about the procedure, whether in written publications or Web sites, should be made available to the patient before the procedure. All questions should be answered and an informed consent form should be completed in advance of the day of the procedure; if informed consent before the procedure is impractical, appropriate modifications can be made (see full discussion on Informed Consent in the next section).

Open-access gastrointestinal endoscopy allows a procedure to be scheduled without meeting a gastroenterologist beforehand. Time and cost considerations have made this format popular recently. Ten years ago 8 million colonoscopies were performed in the United States. With the popularization of this procedure and the fact that screening for colon cancer saves lives, open access for screening examinations would seem to be an efficient model. Patients are busy and do not want to miss work for a "routine" preprocedure visit. Economic pressures and job insecurity have prompted many patients to explain that their employer allows them to miss a day of work for the examination, but not an additional day "just to meet the doctor." Despite attempts to explain that an initial encounter is more than a social nicety, patients often resist the added expense in time and money invested in a preprocedure visit.

With patients scheduling their procedure without a preprocedure consult, the office staff has an even greater responsibility to ensure that the patient understands the procedure and the preparation.

- A list of medications with careful attention to anticoagulation must be obtained before the procedure, with careful instructions on how and when the patient's regular medications should be held or administered.
- If a primary physician can be contacted before the procedure, the endoscopist will gain a more secure insight into the patient's general medical condition. Patients often have several specialists rendering care, making it essential for the endoscopist to understand the patient's general medical condition.

INFORMED CONSENT

Before any procedure, physicians are obligated to obtain "informed consent," which entails explaining the procedure, listing the benefits and risks involved in the procedure, and offering available alternatives. Patients are offered an opportunity to ask questions before starting the procedure. While all attempts are made to assure the patient that their procedure will be without complication, the potential dangers of a procedure and what might happen were there to be an adverse event should be carefully explained. If complications were to occur and the physician has documented that such a discussion took place before the procedure itself, a case of malpractice litigation may even be avoided. Patients are more trusting when they understand and actively participate in the procedure by signing this document as the first step in the process. A study by Robinson illustrated the limitations of informed consent, wherein he recorded his discussion of the potential risks involved in open heart surgery with a patient before surgery, only to have the patient deny ever hearing any of the life-threatening complications when interviewed after the surgery.[4]

ANESTHESIA

Although some procedures can be performed without sedation or analgesics, most patients receive some form of anesthesia for upper endoscopy and colonoscopy, and other endoscopic procedures. Rarely, a patient may be particularly stoic and able to tolerate various degrees of discomfort. Conscious sedation, defined as the use of intravenous drugs to produce a state of depressed consciousness, has been the standard of practice during the performance of endoscopy since the 1970s. This form of moderate anesthesia allows for protective reflexes to be maintained, permits the patient to independently maintain an airway, and enables the patient to preserve appropriate responses to physical or verbal stimulation.

Benzodiazepine Plus Opioid

Historically, a combination of benzodiazepine with an opioid was the most popular sedative agent. The physician and a nurse or endoscopy assistant would monitor the patient's respiratory status while the blood pressure and pulse rate were observed or, in some cases, recorded. Though popular, this drug combination was by no means ideal. The combination can cause respiratory depression, requiring a reduction in dosage. Less medication means less sedation, and patients may be uncomfortable and unable to tolerate the procedure. Doses of anesthesia may need to be limited in patients with multiple medical problems, such as cardiopulmonary disease, cardiomyopathy, or cirrhosis. In a recent survey of endoscopy complications, the 2 factors associated with an increased risk of cardiorespiratory complications were the combined use of a benzodiazepine and an opioid for conscious sedation and performance of an emergent procedure.[5]

Propofol

There has been a major shift to the use of propofol for endoscopic procedures worldwide. Propofol is an ideal agent for endoscopy because of its rapid onset of action and its short half-life. Within 20 to 30 seconds the patient is adequately sedated in a state of moderate to deep sedation, and a procedure can begin. An additional dose can be administered as needed during the procedure to maintain an adequate level of sedation. Most gastroenterologists are not adequately trained in airway management, and should only use propofol with an anesthesiologist or a nurse anesthetist nearby. Whereas some have argued that propofol is a safe agent and can be used by the nonanesthesiologist in an outpatient setting, most surgeons prefer to have an anesthesiologist administer the drug.[6] Many endoscopists work with an anesthesiologist who administers the anesthetic and records the vital signs during the procedure. The added cost is offset by the added safety and comfort of the patient.

Complications of Anesthesia

Complications of anesthesia historically were related to oversedation, particularly in patients with underlying comorbidities. Vasovagal episodes, nausea, and vomiting were not unusual. Midazolam became a popular agent because the local burning sensation and thrombophlebitis at the injection site that accompanied diazepam was virtually eliminated. Midazolam was also a better anamnestic agent than diazepam. Reversal agents such as naloxone and flumazenil were popular in endoscopy suites because when administered they offered a shorter recovery period. However, warnings that these agents have a shorter half-life than the sedative and narcotics themselves made them less attractive for routine use.

Monitoring During Endoscopy

Monitoring during endoscopy should include blood pressure, pulse rate, and oxygen saturation, and should be recorded at baseline, regular intervals, and finally on recovery before discharge. The American Association of Anesthesiology has developed guidelines for the use of anesthesia by the nonanesthesiologist, and recommends that for moderate sedation there should be a trained individual in the room whose responsibility is to monitor the patient's status throughout the procedure.[7] If the level of sedation is beyond conscious sedation the person monitoring the patient should have no other responsibilities, and another person will be needed to assist during the procedure. It is further recommended that an individual with advanced life support skills be available for patients receiving moderate sedation.

Supplemental Oxygen Administration

The routine use of supplemental oxygen is controversial. Although nasal oxygen may reduce the frequency of hypoxemia, some believe it provides a false sense of security and should be administered only when hypoxemia cannot be corrected by jaw thrust or simple airway management. Others maintain that prevention of hypoxemia with supplemental oxygen is preferable to correcting it once it occurs, and that preoxygenation or supplemental oxygen should be used in all high-risk patients undergoing endoscopy. No studies prove that supplemental oxygen should be administered routinely.[8]

POSTPROCEDURE

After the procedure a patient should be in a monitored area until regaining consciousness. Once the nurse, endoscopist, or anesthesiologist determines it is safe for the patient to walk, he or she can be brought to a general waiting area. Before discharge from the office the patient and physician should sit down and have a face-to-face discussion regarding the findings, appropriate follow-up, or any change in medications. A written postprocedure document should be signed by the patient and placed into the permanent record. A written set of postprocedure instructions should be given to the patient and explained. Particular attention to the prohibition of driving for at least 12 hours after the procedure should be emphasized. Particularly after receiving propofol as a single agent, the patient often feels no sedation effect after an hour; nevertheless, the patient should be clearly warned not to drive a car.

A follow-up call by the endoscopist or staff should be made within 24 to 48 hours after the procedure to document the patient's condition. During the conversation the patient should be reminded to call back within an appropriate time to review the results if specimens had been taken for pathologic examination. If a follow-up procedure is indicated, the appointment can be made during the follow-up call. This telephone interaction should be made part of the patient's record.

COMPLICATIONS IN ENDOSCOPY

Considering the number of procedures done in the United States, the low complication rate is testament to the careful training required and vigilance engendered by the national gastroenterological organizations and facility certification. It is generally accepted that the published complication rates are low estimates. While bleeding, perforation and major cardiopulmonary problems are easily identified, and other often-reported complications such as missed lesions are likely underreported. Not all adverse reactions are the same; some are merely an inconvenience while others will have life-altering implications.[9]

As with any complication, the patient and family should be told exactly what has happened and what steps will be taken to correct the problem. Failure to communicate with the patient and the family is the principal reason for malpractice litigation against the practitioner. The physician should explain to the patient and family what has occurred without transmitting a sense of guilt. No attempt at cover-up is acceptable. A professional and caring demeanor should dominate the interaction with the patient and family, who must be assured that all steps will be taken to secure the well-being of the patient. If surgery is indicated, they must be assured that the gastroenterologist will work in tandem with the surgeon and that the patient will be followed daily as needed. A patient feels vulnerable after an unexpected event and easily feels abandoned unless reassured by the practitioner with whom they have a relationship and, possibly, a sense of trust.

COMPLICATIONS UNRELATED TO PERFORMANCE OF THE PROCEDURE

Complications can occur even before the beginning of the procedure. Patients may stop their routine medications and become ill as a result. Diabetics may become ill owing to the rapid change in their nutrition intake the day before and on the day of their procedure. Careful monitoring of their blood glucose levels is important. Some may take the cathartics incorrectly and develop electrolyte imbalance, dehydration, or volume overload. Renal complications have also been reported with magnesium-containing cathartics. Patients with inflammatory bowel disease can worsen their underlying disease with some cathartics. Discussion with their primary physician may be helpful in avoiding these complications.

Infection

Given the types of procedures that gastroenterologists perform, one might expect that infection would be a common complication. Surprisingly, the rate of transmission of infection related to endoscopy is extremely low. The often quoted rate is approximately 1 in 2 million procedures, a number based on data from more than 20 years ago. Reprocessing of endoscopes has become standardized with guidelines from multiple societies, and these rigorous standards have contributed to the maintenance of a low infection rate.[10] The crucial steps to be followed after every procedure are:

1. Cleaning
2. Rinsing
3. Disinfection
4. Rinsing
5. Drying
6. Storage

Manual cleaning includes rinsing and wiping the scope immediately after use. All removable parts are placed in detergents. Channels must be flushed and brushed repeatedly. Manual cleaning has been shown to reduce bacterial burden dramatically. High-level disinfection is achieved through total immersion of the endoscope in a liquid chemical germicide. Most offices reprocess endoscopes in automated reprocessing machines, but these are no substitute for manual cleaning. Meticulous attention must be paid to routine cleaning to avoid transmission of infection. Reports of pathogen transmission from endoscopy have been the result of a breach in following accepted protocol. Automated endoscope reprocessors are cleared by the Food and Drug Administration for high-level disinfection (HLD) of flexible endoscopes when used according to manufacturer's recommendations. All currently available systems are labeled for HLD following manual washing, as outlined by the Society for Gastrointestinal Nurses and Associates.

Although automated, brushless washing of endoscope channels represents a potentially significant advancement, the Technology Committee of the American Society for Gastrointestinal Endoscopy (ASGE) emphasizes the existing multi-society guidelines and other international standards, all of which highlight the importance of manual washing and brushing for the overall efficacy of HLD. The redundancy achieved by adding an automated washing step following manual washing can undoubtedly provide an extra level of safety. All currently used machines in the United States are labeled specifically for use only after manual washing with mechanical brushing. Diligence in application of all steps of washing and disinfection remains paramount in the safe delivery of endoscopic services. The ASGE warns that until further studies become available, mechanical cleaning should always be performed before using an automatic endoscope reprocessor.[11]

Transient bacteremia as a result of diagnostic upper gastrointestinal endoscopy has been reported at rates as high as 8%, but the frequency of infectious endocarditis and other clinical sequelae is extremely low. American Heart Association and ASGE guidelines do not recommend antibiotic prophylaxis solely to prevent bacterial endocarditis.[12]

In 1997 a group in France reported the first documented case of hepatitis C virus transmitted via endoscopy.[13] The report described several breaches in instrument and accessory reprocessing. The endoscope is not the only source of potential infection. The anesthesiologist was the vector of hepatitis C transmission in several outbreaks nationwide. A case familiar to the author involved an anesthesiologist who reused multidose vials of propofol, despite the manufacturer's warning not to use the same vial for more than 1 patient. When a patient reported her own case of hepatitis C to the Department of Health, her source was traced back to the office where she had a routine screening colonoscopy several weeks before her acute illness. The anesthesiologist had performed multiple procedures in the office after an patient positive for hepatitis C virus had undergone a procedure. Reusing the multidose vials allowed the virus to spread from that first patient to several patients thereafter. This sad story has yet to play out in the courts, which will need to address the relationship that exists between the anesthesiologist and the gastroenterologist.

The importance of care and vigilance in rendering endoscopic services in the office setting cannot be overemphasized. The community will hold the physician responsible for maintaining "hospital level" care in the office setting. Centers for Disease Control and Prevention guidelines for universal precautions have been in place since 1985, but compliance with these recommendations may be less than ideal. No excuse will be accepted if an infection results from a breach in established reprocessing standards or if one occurs because guidelines have been disregarded. Disposable accessories offer major advantages of simplicity, sterility, and reduced labor cost for reprocessing, adding only slightly to the overall cost per procedure.

Perforation

Perhaps the most feared complication is perforation during or after a procedure. Although the incidence of perforation is very low, such an untoward event can occur even in the hands of a skilled endoscopist. Perforations during colonoscopy can occur, particularly in someone who has had previous abdominal or pelvic surgery. The adhesed bowel causes fixation, which may not offer the expected "give" during intubation and which can contribute to an unexpected perforation. These perforations occur more commonly in the sigmoid colon. Usually this complication is identified shortly after the procedure when the sedation wears off and the patient complains of abdominal pain. If perforation is suspected an immediate radiograph should be obtained if possible, and surgical consultation sought. Transport to the hospital is indicated, and appropriate intervention should be arranged.

Bleeding

Significant bleeding after upper endoscopy is rare. Minimum platelet counts considered safe for upper endoscopy have not been established; even in patients with thrombocytopenia, bleeding is unusual.[14] With the exception of the anticoagulated patient or one with portal hypertension, major upper gastrointestinal bleeding after upper endoscopy and biopsy is rare.

Hemorrhage after colonoscopy is usually associated with polypectomy; major bleeding after mucosal biopsy is rare. Bleeding after polypectomy of a pedunculated polyp or a sessile lesion can be immediate or be delayed by several days. Large studies estimate the incidence of bleeding to range from 1 to 6 per 1000 colonoscopies.[15] Patients often forget to discontinue daily aspirin despite multiple warnings. On the morning of their procedure, particularly after purging themselves, they are sometimes too embarrassed to admit that they had forgotten to stop their aspirin 5 to 7 days before their examination, which will likely contribute to postpolypectomy hemorrhage. In cases of bleeding at the stalk site, clips or bands can be applied to the oozing site. In the absence of a coagulopathy, most bleeding will spontaneously stop but may require inpatient monitoring for several days.

Cardiopulmonary

Cardiopulmonary complications range from events of little clinical significance such as minor fluctuations in oxygen saturation or heart rate, to serious complications including respiratory arrest, cardiac arrhythmias, myocardial infarction, and shock. In one study that used a research database, cardiopulmonary complications occurred in 0.9% of procedures. Transient hypoxemia occurred in 230 per 100,000 cases, but prolonged hypoxemia occurred in only 0.78 per 100,000 colonoscopies. Although the data may underestimate the acute complications because of underreporting, cardiopulmonary complications are unusual in patients without multiple comorbid disease.[16]

Missed Lesions

A great deal of attention has been devoted to the problem of missed lesions during endoscopic procedures. Many theories have been offered to understand why lesions might not be identified, including rapid endoscopic withdrawal time and inadequate quality of preparation of the colon, and flat or depressed lesions that may not be apparent on even a careful examination.[17] What most experts agree is that, even in skilled hands, from 4% to 10% of lesions larger than 10 mm might not be detected.

Death

In a 2010 review of colonoscopy complications based on prospective studies and retrospective analyses of large clinical or administrative databases, there were 128 deaths reported among 371,099 colonoscopies, for an unweighted pooled death rate of 0.03%.[16] Death from endoscopy is almost always related to comorbid disease, and will call into question the advisability of performing the procedure in an office.

DOCUMENTATION

The endoscopist's report can be formatted by handwritten notes, preprinted forms, computer databases, or individually typed reports. Careful attention must be paid if an electronic report has preformatted sections, because the final report may contain gross inaccuracies. For example, if the cecum was not reached but the body of the "drop down" states that the cecum and landmarks were identified, the internal inconsistencies will suggest sloppy and inaccurate care during the procedure. Hurried notes will suggest hurried incomplete care.[18]

Reports should include the indications for the procedure and any additional special issues. If an unexpected complication were to occur in a patient whose indication for undertaking the risk was not substantiated, the physician will and should have some accountability. Defense of potential litigation will also be more difficult if the procedure was not indicated.

The report should indicate the method of anesthesia and the patient's general tolerance of the procedure. If an anesthesiologist is present, an additional full anesthesia record should be part of the endoscopy report.

All reports should clearly describe the findings and any abnormalities or unusual aspects of the examination. If biopsy specimens were taken, their location and number should be noted. A diagnosis should be recorded and a plan for further management or follow-up treatment, and the need for further procedures, should be recorded. The report should be sent to the referring physician. Serious findings should be directly communicated to the other physicians involved in the patient's care. If the procedure was prompted by self-referral or was performed in a patient from another state or even another country, a copy of the endoscopy report should be sent to the patient directly.

SUMMARY

Office endoscopy is an accepted safe alternative to in-hospital care. Attention to detail will help to ensure that the vast majority of procedures will be successfully completed without incident. An office setting offers advantages for the patient and the endoscopist. Patients will be cared for in a familiar surrounding by staff they likely have interacted with at a prior visit. The office should be able to personalize the care and minimize what might be a stressful and anxiety-provoking visit. The physician will be able to work at his or her own pace with staff that knows exactly how each procedure will be performed. The physician should assure the patient that in the office every detail has been carefully scrutinized for the patient's care and safety. Unexpected events can occur despite the safest environment and in the best of hands. Recognizing a complication and taking all steps to rectify the situation in a timely and appropriate fashion is important for patients' well-being. The safety of patients depends on a well-designed infrastructure and a staff that works together harmoniously, a facility that calls for constant support and attention to detail and not simply a skilled endoscopist.

REFERENCES

1. Brandt LJ. Patients' attitudes and apprehensions about endoscopy: how to calm troubled waters. Am J Gastroenterol 2001;96:280–4.
2. ASGE Standards of Practice Committee, Jain R, Ikenberry SO, Anderson MA, et al. Minimum staffing requirements for the performance of GI endoscopy. Gastrointest Endosc 2010;72(3):469–70.
3. ASGE Standards of Practice Committee, Levy MJ, Anderson MA, Baron TH, et al. Position statement on routine laboratory testing before endoscopic procedures. Gastrointest Endosc 2008;68(5):827–32.
4. Robinson G, Merav A. Recall of patients post-operatively. Ann Thorac Surg 1976;22:209–12.
5. Arrowsmith JB, Gerstman BB, Fleischer DE, et al. Results from the American Society for Gastrointestinal Endoscopy/U.S. Food and Drug Administration collaborative study on complication rates and drug use during gastrointestinal endoscopy. Gastrointest Endosc 1991;37:421–7.
6. Cohen LB, Dubovsky AN, Aisenberg J. Propofol for endoscopic sedation: a protocol for safe and effective administration by the gastroenterologist. Gastrointest Endosc 2003;58(5):725–32.
7. American Society of Anesthesiologists Task Force on Sedation and Analgesia by Non-Anesthesiologists. Guidelines for sedation and analgesia by non-anesthesiologists. Anesthesiology 2002;96:1004–17.
8. Bell GD. Who is for supplemental oxygen [editorial]. Gastrointest Endosc 1992;38:514–6.
9. Cotton P, Eisen G, Aabakken L. A lexicon for endoscopic adverse events; report of an ASGE workshop. Gastrointest Endosc 2010;71(3):446–54.

10. Multi-society guidelines for reprocessing flexible gastrointestinal endoscope. Gastrointest Endosc 2003;58:1–8.

11. American Society for Gastrointestinal Endoscopy. ASGE reprocessing of flexible gastrointestinal endoscopes. Gastrointest Endosc 1996;43: 540–6.

12. Banerjee S, Shen B, Baron TH, et al. Antibiotic prophylaxis for GI endoscopy. Gastrointest Endosc 2008;67:791–8.

13. Bronowicki JP, Venard V, Botte C. Patient to patient transmission of hepatitis c virus during colonoscopy. N Engl J Med 1997;337:237–40.

14. Anderson MA, Ben-Menachem T, Gan SI, et al. Management of antithrombotic agents for endoscopic procedures. Gastrointest Endosc 2009;70:1060–70.

15. Ko CW, Dominitz JA. Complications of colonoscopy: magnitude and management. Gastrointest Endosc Clin N Am 2010;20:659–71.

16. ASGE Standards of Practice Committee, Fisher DA, Maple JT, Ben-Menachem T, et al. Complications of colonoscopy. Gastrointest Endosc 2011;74(4):745–52.

17. Pabby A, Schoen RE, Weissfeld JL, et al. Analysis of colorectal cancer occurrence during surveillance colonoscopy in the dietary Polyp Prevention Trial. Gastrointest Endosc 2005;61:385–91.

18. Cotton P, Saxton JW, Finkelstein MM. Avoiding medicolegal complications. Gastrointest Endosc Clin N Am 2007;17:197–207.

Hypothermia and Hyperthermia in the Ambulatory Surgical Patient

Michael Hernandez, MD, Thomas W. Cutter, MD, MEd,
Jeffrey L. Apfelbaum, MD*

KEYWORDS

- Hypothermia • Hyperthermia • Ambulatory surgical patient • Malignant hyperthermia treatment

KEY POINTS

- Anesthetic medications and techniques can disrupt the thermoregulatory process in surgical patients. Temperature monitoring is essential in patients to preserve normothermia.
- Even mild hypothermia may cause bleeding, myocardial events, infection, and postoperative pain.
- Untreated, malignant hyperthermia leads to morbidity or death. The perioperative team must be familiar with its diagnosis and prepared with a treatment plan.
- Immediate care for malignant hyperthermia demands the ready availability of a cart stocked with dantrolene, diluent, and adjunctive treatment drugs.
- A patient with malignant hyperthermia requires continued postoperative care and, if necessary, transfer to an acute care facility.

Homeotherms, including humans, are able to maintain a relatively constant temperature despite variations in their thermal environment. We normally maintain a narrow thermoregulatory threshold range of approximately 0.2°C, and little change in core temperature is required to trigger compensatory mechanisms to either cool or warm our core temperature back to normothermia. This article focuses on the mechanisms and consequences of hypothermia and hyperthermia in the surgical patient and reviews techniques to prevent and treat these conditions.

NORMAL REGULATORY MECHANISMS

Maintaining core temperature is a complex process. Initially, the hypothalamus was believed to be primarily responsible for temperature regulation, but it has since become clear that spinal cord pathways, abdominal organs, and skin surface temperature contribute to the activation of autonomic thermoregulatory mechanisms, including shivering, vasoconstriction, sweating, and vasodilation.[1] The complexity and multiple locations of thermoregulatory control help explain why a wide range of anesthetic medications and techniques can disrupt normal temperature. Vasoconstriction and shivering take place when the core temperature decreases lower than the lower limit of the thermoregulatory threshold, whereas sweating and vasodilation represent a central response to a core temperature that exceeds the upper limit of the thermoregulatory threshold. Peripheral temperature is usually cooler than the core by 2° to 4°C, with the gradient maintained by peripheral vasoconstriction of arteriovenous shunts.[1] Core heat is conserved and heat dissipation to the environment is prevented to maintain normothermia in an unanesthetized person, but thermoregulation and other processes are often disrupted in an anesthetized patient.

HYPOTHERMIA

Hypothermia is defined as a core body temperature less than 36°C.[2] Despite an effective

Department of Anesthesia and Critical Care, The University of Chicago Medicine, 5841 S. Maryland Avenue, MC 4028 Chicago, IL 60637, USA
* Corresponding author.
E-mail address: jeffa@dacc.uchicago.edu

Clin Plastic Surg 40 (2013) 429–438
http://dx.doi.org/10.1016/j.cps.2013.04.015
0094-1298/13/$ – see front matter © 2013 Elsevier Inc. All rights reserved.

homeothermic thermoregulatory system, patients can become hypothermic perioperatively, when the thermoregulatory threshold is widened under the effects of sedation, general anesthesia, or regional anesthesia (**Fig. 1**).[3]

General Anesthesia

Anesthetic agents disrupt a patient's normal thermoregulatory mechanisms in different ways,[4–7] including the loss of behavioral mechanisms (ie, putting on a jacket when cold) because of loss of consciousness to inhibition of autonomic responses, such as shivering and vasoconstriction (**Fig. 2**). The development of hypothermia during general anesthesia can be described in 3 phases (**Fig. 3**).

First Phase (Redistribution)

The first or redistribution phase of core temperature heat loss occurs shortly after induction of general anesthesia (**Fig. 4**). Peripheral vasodilation transfers core body heat to the periphery and subsequently to the environment. With general anesthesia, a core temperature decline fails to trigger normal thermoregulatory vasoconstriction (ie, the body's thermostat is reset to defend a temperature <37°C). As a result, the normal core/peripheral

temperature gradient becomes smaller, with greater heat loss to the environment. Most of the heat loss during a general anesthetic from core/peripheral redistribution occurs within the first hour of the anesthetic and, in the absence of active warming, the patient's core temperature can decline 1°C to 1.5°C.[8] Redistribution contributes to approximately 80% of heat loss in the first hour, but is not the only contributor.[8] General anesthesia can decrease metabolic heat production by approximately one-third, and exposure to a cool ambient environment, administration of cool intravenous fluids, and the application of cool skin-cleaning solutions can result in up to 5% of additional first-phase heat loss.

Second Phase (Linear)

Without active warming, core temperature declines linearly during the second hour, resulting in the loss of another 1°C to 2°C of core temperature. Core to peripheral heat redistribution contributes only 40% of heat loss during the second phase.[8] Most heat loss during the second phase occurs as a result of decreased metabolic heat production in the setting of cool intravenous fluid administration and the exposure of a large body surface area or large wounds. Heat is lost via radiation,

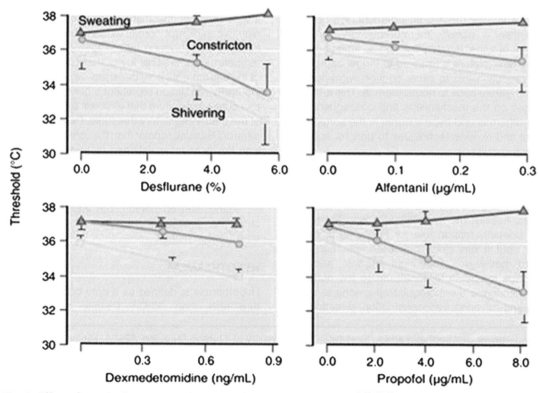

Fig. 1. Effect of anesthetic agents on thermoregulation. (*Data from* Refs.[5,12,47,48])

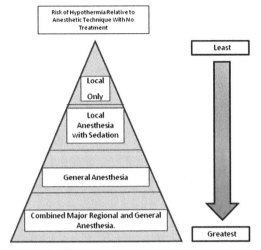

Fig. 2. Risk of hypothermia.

convection, evaporation, and conduction, and outpaces the diminished metabolic heat production during a general anesthetic.

Plateau Phase

The third phase of intraoperative hypothermia is the plateau phase, typically during the third hour of general anesthesia.[9] The plateau phase is characterized by a relatively constant core temperature even with increased surgical time. Heat loss continues, but core temperature is preserved by the restoration of the core/periphery temperature gradient, at a lower temperature, and the activation of autonomic thermoregulatory mechanisms.[10] Plateau phase core temperatures typically reach between 34°C and 35°C.

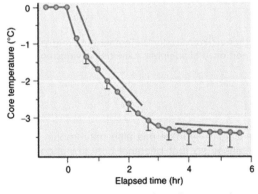

Fig. 3. Phases of temperature loss. (*From* Sessler DI. Temperature regulation and monitoring. In: Miller RD, editor. Miller's anesthesia. 7th edition. Philadelphia: Churchill Livingstone; 2010. p. 1538; with permission.)

Regional Anesthesia

A major regional anesthetic causes vasodilation and the loss of afferent signaling to the hypothalamus within the affected area. Anesthetized tissue not only loses heat rapidly but also loses heat without signals to the central regulatory system that would activate vasoconstriction and shivering. As a result, patients may subjectively feel warm despite hypothermia (**Fig. 5**). With vasodilation, redistribution of heat loss is similar to that in the first phase of a general anesthetic and in the case of epidural blockade, core temperature decreases 0.8°C ± 0.3°C during the first hour.[11] Heat loss from redistribution is less than during general anesthesia because part of the body is spared vasodilation, but redistribution remains the primary mechanism of heat loss during regional anesthesia. In the linear phase, heat loss through radiation, convection, evaporation, and conduction may still exceed metabolic heat production, and core temperature may continue to decrease over hours 1 to 3 of the anesthetic. A patient under the influence of a prolonged major regional anesthetic (eg, an epidural block) may not achieve a thermal steady state or plateau phase. Vasoconstriction and shivering do not return during regional anesthesia (as they do during general anesthesia), because of peripheral blockade of the anesthetized area.

Local Anesthesia

Infiltration of a local anesthetic that does not result in major conduction blockade does not affect thermoregulation perioperatively, but many patients who undergo a procedure with infiltration of a local anesthetic also may receive intravenous sedation or analgesia. Opioids and propofol, which disrupt normal thermoregulation,[5,12] put patients at risk for perioperative hypothermia. Midazolam is unique among anesthetic agents, because it does not seem to appreciably alter thermoregulation.[13] The risk of hypothermia in sedated patients should be considered even if most of the analgesia is provided by infiltration of local anesthetics.

Consequences of Hypothermia

Mild hypothermia can have deleterious effects perioperatively on coagulation,[14] wound healing and infection,[15,16] patient satisfaction, recovery time,[17] drug metabolism, and the rate of perioperative myocardial events. Although controversy persists regarding the clinical significance of coagulopathy that results from mild hypothermia, the investigators of 1 meta-analysis concluded that

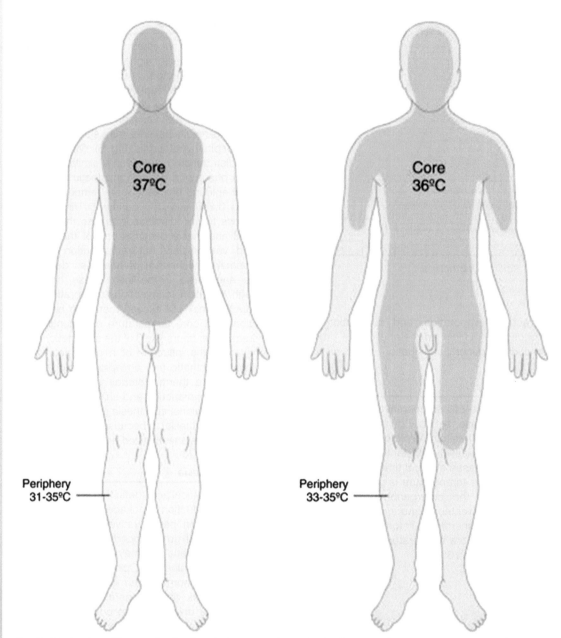

Fig. 4. Mechanism of heat redistribution during general anesthesia. (*From* Sessler DI. Temperature regulation and monitoring. In: Miller RD, editor. Miller's anesthesia. 7th edition. Philadelphia: Churchill Livingstone; 2010. p. 1538; with permission.)

mild hypothermia, even a decrease of less than 1°C from core normothermia, is sufficient to increase procedural blood loss by 16%.[14] Mild hypothermia is believed to increase the risk of wound infection by several mechanisms. Vasoconstriction reduces blood flow to wounds, lessening subcutaneous oxygen tension locally and predisposing to wound infection and delayed healing.[18] Hypothermia also may impair immune defenses so that bacterial contamination results in infection.[19] A 2°C core temperature decline from normothermia tripled the rate of wound infection after colon resection,[15] so maintaining normothermia perioperatively has the potential to decrease the chances of a surgical wound infection.[16]

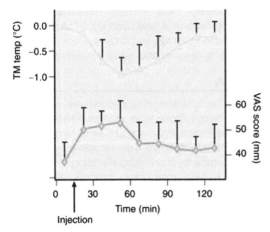

Fig. 5. Temperature decline and patient temperature visual analog temperature scale (VAS) after epidural anesthesia. (*Data from* Sessler DI, Ponte J. Shivering during epidural anesthesia. Anesthesiology 1990;72: 816–21.)

Hypothermia also may affect myocardial events. Although metabolic demand from shivering may have a small effect on myocardial events, increased release of catecholamines[20] in the hypothermic patient may predispose to myocardial events. Patients with hypothermia of less than 2°C had a greater than double risk of a myocardial event than did a normothermic group.[21]

Mild hypothermia also slows the metabolism of many drugs typically used as anesthetic agents. Hypothermia alters the pharmacokinetics of medications such as propofol, neuromuscular blocking agents, and even the volatile anesthetic agents.[20] A decrease in core temperature of 3°C increased propofol plasma concentrations and prolonged duration of neuromuscular blockade with atracurium.[22] A hypothermic patient may suffer from delayed awakening and a longer duration of neuromuscular blockade. Mildly hypothermic patients may increase metabolic heat production by shivering postoperatively, an unpleasant sensation for most people and even more so when postoperative wounds are fresh. As a result, postoperative hypothermia may contribute to patient dissatisfaction and prolong the recovery period.[17,23]

The consequences of mild perioperative hypothermia have led to policies to encourage the maintenance of perioperative normothermia. The basic monitoring standards of the American Society of Anesthesiologists state that "every patient receiving anesthesia shall have temperature monitored when clinically significant changes in body temperature are intended, anticipated or suspected."[24] An American Society of Plastic Surgeons task force on patient safety advised that office-based facilities have temperature monitoring equipment and the ability to adjust temperature and actively warm patients.[25] Facilities that do not have such capabilities should accept patients only for procedures expected to last 2 hours or less that involve no more than 20% of the body surface area. The standards of the Surgical Care Improvement Project require that patients have at least 1 documented temperature of 36°C within the 30 minutes before or 15 minutes after the documented anesthesia end time or the documented use of active warming intraoperatively.[26] The Center for Medicare and Medicaid Services has also adopted this criterion for reimbursement. Thus, the prevention of perioperative hypothermia not only optimizes patient outcomes, but is used as a metric for institutional performance.

Measurement Devices and Techniques

Maintaining normothermia and treating hypothermia require reliable and accurate core temperature monitoring, which is not always easy to obtain. An invasive pulmonary artery catheter provides accurate monitoring of core temperature but is impractical for most patients, especially in the ambulatory setting. The direct application of a temperature probe to the tympanic membrane provides a good monitor of core temperature,[27] but more readily available infrared tympanic temperature monitors fail to reliably approximate core temperature unless properly placed directly in front of the tympanic membrane.[28] Nasopharyngeal measurement also reasonably approximates core temperature.[29] Distal measurement of esophageal temperature is a good method of temperature monitoring used by anesthesiologists during a general anesthetic, but for a nonintubated patient, esophageal temperature probes are impractical. Additional measurement sites include the rectum and bladder, but temperature values can be affected by local factors, including urine output. In an ambulatory setting, rectal measurement of temperature can be a good option for patients who undergo a lower body regional anesthetic with attendant perineal blockade.

Cutaneous temperature monitoring may be used as a proxy for core temperature measurement but is better suited for trending than for accuracy. Axillary temperature monitoring works best when the temperature probe is placed over the patient's axillary artery and the corresponding arm is tucked beside the torso.[30,31] Adhesive liquid crystal thermometer strips can be useful for core temperature monitoring if placed properly. The skin of the forehead is typically 2°C cooler than the core, and this relationship is well maintained as core temperature changes.[32] Even if an accurate core temperature reading is elusive, monitoring can at least identify a trend of cooling or heating that threatens normothermia.

Preventing Hypothermia

The 2 methods of maintaining a patient's temperature perioperatively are passive and active warming. Passive techniques prevent the loss of heat without specifically adding any heat to the system. Blankets, surgical drapes, and passively humidified respiratory gases are examples of passive warming. Although passive warming can limit heat loss, it has not been shown to prevent hypothermia.[33]

Unlike passive techniques, active warming adds external heat. Radiant heat lamps, higher ambient (room) temperatures, forced air blankets, and fluid warmers are examples of active warming methods. Forced air warmers are the most commonly used active warming devices. Comparisons of forced air warming devices with passive devices such as cotton blankets and reflective blankets have shown that forced air blankets are superior for maintaining normothermia.[33–35] To be effective, a forced air blanket must let warmed air circulate and must be in contact with the patient's body. Peripheral heat content gain during the preoperative phase has been shown to diminish heat loss during the redistribution of heat from the core to the periphery in phase 1 of the intraoperative phase.[35]

Administration of intravenous fluids at room temperature can lower body temperature by 0.25°C per liter,[36] but warmed intravenous fluids can help prevent perioperative hypothermia. The combination of forced air warming and warmed intravenous fluid administration (average 6 L) has been suggested to be superior to forced air warming alone, preventing perioperative hypothermia in major surgery.[37]

Fluids used for irrigation and tumescent infiltration can also contribute to the development of perioperative hypothermia. A comparison of lipoplasty patients treated with cool (27°C) versus heated (37°C) tumescent solution without additional active warming showed both groups to be hypothermic at the end of the 3.5-hour procedure.[38] The group who received heated tumescent solution did maintain a higher mean core temperature (35.7°C) than the group who received cool tumescence (34.9°C), showing that warming infiltration fluids does not prevent hypothermia without other active measures. Also, procedures that require large amounts of irrigation fluid or tumescent solution often result in exposure of greater patient body surface area, which may accelerate patient heat loss perioperatively. Thus, warming solutions for irrigation or infiltration are best used in combination with other active warming techniques, such as forced air warming devices and warm intravenous fluids.

Summary

Most patients undergoing procedures with anesthesia, except those who receive infiltration with local anesthetics only, are at risk of hypothermia. Even mild hypothermia may negatively affect patient outcome by increasing bleeding, myocardial events, wound infections, postoperative pain, and recovery time. The risks of perioperative hypothermia must be recognized, and we must be vigilant in detecting, treating, and preventing it (**Box 1**). Temperature monitoring is essential to the preservation of patient normothermia. Monitoring is critical in procedures involving major regional anesthetics, because physicians may be unable to detect and patients unable to react to hypothermia. Maintenance of normothermia is best accomplished with the use of forced air warming devices over a sufficient period to minimize loss of core heat. A coordinated effort during the preoperative, intraoperative, and postoperative care phases is essential for preventing hypothermia.

HYPERTHERMIA

Perioperative hyperthermia results from excessive heat added to the patient, such as may ensue from overzealous attempts to prevent hypothermia, or from endogenous heat production in a wide range of medical conditions, including sepsis, hypothalamic dysfunction, thyroid dysfunction, substance abuse, neuromuscular disorders, and malignant hyperthermia (MH). This section focuses on MH.

MH is a unique condition associated with commonly used anesthetic agents, which may cause

---

Box 1
Risk factors for hypothermia

Extremes of age (geriatric and neonatal patients)

Combined general and regional anesthesia

Low ambient OR temperature

Low preoperative patient peripheral temperature

Thin body habitus

High blood loss

High-exposure surgery (ie, burns)

Data from Macario A, Dexter F. What are the most important risk factors for a patient's developing intraoperative hypothermia? Anesth Analg 2002;94: 215–20.

serious morbidity or mortality if left unrecognized or if treatment is delayed. A pharmacogenetic disorder that follows an autosomal-dominant pattern with incomplete penetrance,[39] MH involves the disordered regulation of intracellular calcium, which prolongs and sustains skeletal muscle contraction and causes a hypermetabolic state.

Mechanism of MH and Triggering Agents

Triggering agents of MH are all volatile inhalational anesthetics (eg, sevoflurane) and succinylcholine. Nonvolatile inhalational anesthetics (eg, nitrous oxide) do not trigger MH. Succinylcholine, a depolarizing muscle relaxant commonly used to facilitate tracheal intubation and to treat airway emergencies such as laryngospasm, works differently from nondepolarizing muscle relaxants (eg, cisatracurium and rocuronium). A general anesthetic may include 1 or more triggering agents, making vigilance for MH imperative.

Identification of Susceptible Patients

A history of the signs and symptoms of MH in a patient or a relative during a previous anesthetic can indicate MH susceptibility, but a definitive medical history is often lacking. Patients may simply recall a relative who almost died in the operating room or had some other nonspecific perioperative course. When historical information is vague, the anesthesiologist is left to weigh the risks and benefits of avoiding triggering agents in a patient. It is not uncommon for physicians to dismiss the possibility of MH susceptibility in patients who have had uneventful general anesthetics in the past, but MH susceptibility is a result of many possible genetic mutations, with variable expression, and MH susceptibility cannot be excluded by a history of uneventful general anesthetics.[40]

Preparation for MH

MH is rare, with estimates of 1 in 100,000.[41] It is not uncommon for anesthesiologists to finish their careers without having to manage a case of MH. Although planning and preparing for rare but potentially catastrophic events is difficult, the Malignant Hyperthermia Association of the United States (MHAUS) is a resource for the prevention and treatment of MH. Any location that uses MH-triggering medications must be prepared to diagnose and treat and, if necessary, transfer a patient with MH for intensive care. Although preparation for MH requires costly economic and staff resources, the alternative of a bad outcome for a patient is costlier still.[42]

The American Association for Accreditation of Ambulatory Surgery Facilities (AAAASF) and the Accreditation Association for Ambulatory Health Care (AAAHC) address MH in their requirements for accreditation. The AAAHC refers to a statement from MHAUS that advises that centers in which triggering agents are used should have 36 vials of dantrolene available. The AAAASF directives give a detailed list of supplies, which includes dantrolene (12 vials, with immediate access to 24 more within 15 minutes), MHAUS treatment literature on the MH cart, a plan for transfer of patients to an acute care setting, and regularly documented staff drills and assigned roles during an MH crisis (**Fig. 6**).[43] State regulations regarding MH preparation vary. Local regulations should be verified, because the required minimum number of stocked vials of dantrolene is different from state to state.

Signs of MH

Increased temperature in MH does not necessarily represent the best or earliest indicator of the condition. MH is fundamentally a hypermetabolic state, fueled by the abnormal and prolonged contraction of skeletal muscle, with increased carbon dioxide production secondary to increased metabolism. Excretion levels of carbon dioxide, which is cleared during ventilation, increase on end-tidal monitoring in patients with MH. In 1 review, hypercarbia was the first or only sign of MH at presentation in 38% of 255 patients.[44] Other early indicators included sinus tachycardia (31%) and masseter spasm (20.8%). Rapid temperature increase, or temperature greater than 38.8°C, was the first sign in only 8.2% of the same patient population.

Hypercarbia and sinus tachycardia during general anesthesia are not pathognomonic for MH, so other signs help support the diagnosis. In addition to ventilatory acidosis, a metabolic acidosis, as measured by arterial blood gas, is common. Muscle rigidity also may be present, along with increased plasma creatinine kinase levels from muscle breakdown. Rhabdomyolysis may produce cola-colored urine from myoglobinuria and hyperkalemia, the latter potentially leading to cardiac arrest. Death may also ensue from the extreme acidosis and temperature increase.

Treatment of MH

Effective treatment of an MH crisis requires coordination and swift action. MHAUS has posters and a Web page with detailed treatment algorithms and a 24-hour hotline staffed by experts (**Box 2**). Triggering agents should be discontinued and intravenous dantrolene sodium, which lessens the calcium release that fuels the hypermetabolic state, should be administered as quickly as

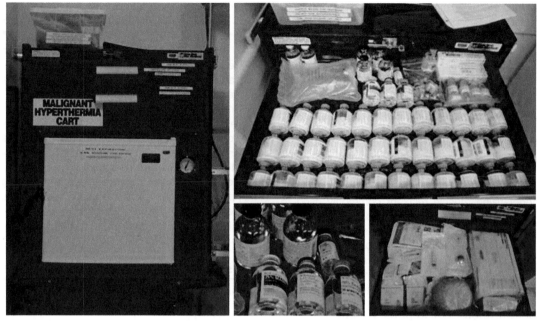

Fig. 6. MH roller cart with vials of dantrolene, diluent, adjunctive drugs (eg, mannitol, sodium bicarbonate, calcium, dextrose), and miscellaneous supplies.

possible.[45] The reconstitution and administration of dantrolene can be labor intensive, and additional personnel should be mobilized to ensure a rapid response. Supportive care includes cooling

---

Box 2
MHAUS MH treatment recommendations

CALL the MH 24-hour hotline (for emergencies only)

- United States: 1+800-644-9737
- Outside the US: 00+1+303-389-1647

Start emergency therapy for MH acute phase treatment

1. Get help. Get dantrolene. Notify surgeon
2. Dantrolene sodium for injection 2.5 mg/kg rapidly IV through large-bore IV, if possible
3. Bicarbonate for metabolic acidosis
4. Cool the patient
5. Dysrhythmias: usually respond to treatment of acidosis and hyperkalemia
6. Hyperkalemia
7. Follow: ETCO$_2$, electrolytes, blood gases, CK, serum myoglobin, core temperature, urine output and color, and coagulation studies

Adapted from Malignant Hyperthermia Association of the United States. Available at: http://www.mhaus.org/healthcare-professionals/ accessed 10/17/2012.

---

of the patient, treating a metabolic acidosis with bicarbonate, monitoring and treating hyperkalemia, and administering diuretics and fluids to maintain urine output. Laboratory tests should include arterial blood gas analysis, creatinine kinase, myoglobin, electrolytes, and coagulation studies.

Transfer to an acute care facility should be considered soon after a diagnosis of MH, particularly if resources for laboratory studies and critical care management are lacking. Arrangements for transfer of patients to an acute care facility are best made in advance, and an agreement should already be in place between an ambulatory surgery center or office surgical suite and an acute care facility equipped to take care of patients in MH crisis. A guide for the transfer of patients with MH from an ambulatory surgery center to an acute care hospital makes several recommendations.[46] A mechanism should exist for rapid mobilization of transport (emergency medical services or otherwise), reliable communication between treating physicians and accepting physicians, and appropriate critical care and dantrolene resources at the receiving hospital.

After successful treatment of the acute phase of an MH crisis, a patient still requires intensive monitoring. MH may recur despite initial dantrolene treatment, and repeat dosing of dantrolene is recommended. Once patients have recovered from an MH crisis, they must be counseled about the diagnosis and its hereditary ramifications. The newly diagnosed MH-susceptible patient should be educated on the condition and the implications for family members.

Summary

There are many reasons why a patient may become hyperthermic in the perioperative period. Most of the time, the patient's comorbidities, such as infection with sepsis, endocrine disorders, and or iatrogenic overheating, are the cause. However, the rapid morbidity and mortality of untreated MH demand that all members of the perioperative team be familiar with the diagnosis and treatment of the condition. The possibility of MH must be considered any time a patient is cared for in a facility housing triggering agents. Even if there is no intent to use succinylcholine or volatile anesthetic agents, the presence of these agents in a facility requires an MH treatment plan. It is also critical to realize that patients with previous uncomplicated exposure to triggering agents may suffer an MH crisis with subsequent exposure to triggering agents. Institutional preparation for MH crises is as important as the education and training of the perioperative team. An MH cart fully stocked with nonexpired dantrolene, diluent, and adjunctive treatment drugs and equipment must always be at the ready in facilities housing triggering agents. Similarly, a plan for the continued care of a patient with MH must be operational at all times. Surgical facilities should have agreements in place for transfer of the patient with MH to an acute care setting with critical care capabilities, when such resources are lacking in the original location. MH is a rare disorder, with potentially catastrophic outcomes. Patient survival without permanent sequelae is possible with prompt diagnosis and treatment. All members of the perioperative team must be prepared to recognize and treat MH.

REFERENCES

1. Kurz A. Physiology of thermoregulation. Best Pract Res Clin Anaesthesiol 2008;22(4):627–44.
2. Sessler DI. Mild perioperative hypothermia. N Engl J Med 1997;336(24):1730–7.
3. Sessler DI. Central thermoregulatory inhibition by general anesthesia. Anesthesiology 1991;75:557–9.
4. Ikeda T, Kim JS, Sessler DI, et al. The volatile anesthetic, isoflurane, alters shivering patterns and reduces maximum shivering intensity. Anesthesiology 1998;88:866–73.
5. Kurz A, Go JC, Sessler DI, et al. The narcotic alfentanil slightly increases the sweating threshold but markedly reduces the vasoconstriction and shivering thresholds. Anesthesiology 1995;83:293–9.
6. Kurz A, Xiong J, Sessler DI, et al. Another volatile anesthetic, desflurane, reduces the gain of thermoregulatory arteriovenous shunt vasoconstriction in humans. Anesthesiology 1995;83:1212–9.
7. Stoen R, Sessler DI. The thermoregulatory threshold is inversely proportional to isoflurane concentration. Anesthesiology 1990;72:822–7.
8. Matsukawa T, Sessler DI, Sessler AM, et al. Heat flow and distribution during induction of general anesthesia. Anesthesiology 1995;83(5):961–7.
9. Kurz A, Sessler DI, Christensen R, et al. Heat balance and distribution during the core temperature plateau in anesthetized humans. Anesthesiology 1995;83:491–9.
10. Belani K, Sessler DI, Sessler AM, et al. Leg heat content continues to decrease during the core temperature plateau in humans. Anesthesiology 1993;78:856–63.
11. Matsukawa T, Sessler DI, Christensen R, et al. Heat flow and distribution during epidural anesthesia. Anesthesiology 1995;83(5):961–7.
12. Matsukawa T, Kurz A, Sessler DI, et al. Propofol linearly reduces the vasoconstriction and shivering thresholds. Anesthesiology 1995;82:1169–80.
13. Kurz A, Sessler DI, Annadata R, et al. Midazolam minimally impairs thermoregulatory control. Anesth Analg 1995;81:393–8.
14. Rajagopalan S, Mascha E, Na J, et al. The effects of mild perioperative hypothermia on blood loss and transfusion requirement: a meta-analysis. Anesthesiology 2008;108:71–7.
15. Kurz A, Sessler DI, Lenhardt R. Perioperative normothermia to reduce the incidence of surgical wound infection and shorten hospitalization. N Engl J Med 1996;334:1209–15.
16. Melling AC, Ali B, Scott EM, et al. Effects of preoperative warming on the incidence of wound infection after clean surgery: a randomized controlled trial. Lancet 2001;358:876–80.
17. Lenhardt R, Marker E, Goll V, et al. Mild intraoperative hypothermia prolongs postanesthetic recovery. Anesthesiology 1997;87:1318–23.
18. Sheffield CW, Sessler DI, Hopf HW, et al. Centrally and locally mediated thermoregulatory responses alter subcutaneous oxygen tension. Wound Repair Regen 1996;4(3):339–45.
19. van Oss CJ, Absolom DR, Moore LL, et al. Effect of temperature on the chemotaxis, phagocytic engulfment, digestion and O_2 consumption of human polymorphonuclear leukocytes. J Reticuloendothel Soc 1980;27:561–5.
20. Kurz A. Thermal care in the perioperative period. Best Pract Res Clin Anaesthesiol 2008;22(1):39–62.
21. Frank SM, Fleisher LA, Breslow MJ, et al. Perioperative maintenance of normothermia reduces the

incidence of morbid cardiac events: a randomized clinical trial. JAMA 1997;277:1127–34.

22. Leslie K, Sessler DI, Bjorksten AR, et al. Mild hypothermia alters propofol pharmacokinetics and increased the duration of action of atracurium. Anesth Analg 1995;80:1007–14.

23. Sessler DI, Rubinstein EH, Moayeri A. Physiological responses to mild perianesthetic hypothermia in humans. Anesthesiology 1999;90:1609–16.

24. ASA Basic Anesthetic Monitoring, Standards For. Available at: http://www.asahq.org/For-Members/Clinical-Information/Standards-Guidelines-and-Statements.aspx. Accessed October 9, 2012.

25. Iverson RE. ASPS task force on patient safety in office-based surgery facilities. Plast Reconstr Surg 2002;110(5):1337–42.

26. Available at: http://www.jointcommission.org/specifications_manual_for_national_hospital_inpatient_quality_measures.aspx. Accessed October 9, 2012.

27. Benzinger M. Tympanic thermometry in surgery and anesthesia. JAMA 1969;209:1207–11.

28. Imamura M, Matsukawa T, Ozaki M, et al. The accuracy and precision of four infrared aural canal thermometers during cardiac surgery. Acta Anaesthesiol Scand 1998;42:1222–6.

29. Cork RC, Vaughan RW, Humphrey LS. Precision and accuracy of intraoperative temperature monitoring. Anesth Analg 1983;62:211–4.

30. Sessler DI. Temperature monitoring and perioperative thermoregulation. Anesthesiology 2008;109:318–38.

31. Lodha R, Mukerji N, Sinha N, et al. Is axillary temperature an appropriate surrogate for core temperature? Indian J Pediatr 2000;67:571–4.

32. Ikeda T, Sessler DI, Marder D, et al. The influence of thermoregulatory vasomotion and ambient temperature variation on the accuracy of core temperature estimates by cutaneous liquid crystal thermometers. Anesthesiology 1997;86:603–12.

33. Ng SF, Oo CS, Loh KH, et al. A comparative study of three warming interventions to determine the most effective in maintaining perioperative normothermia. Anesth Analg 2003;96:171–6.

34. Horn EP, Bein B, Bohm R, et al. The effect of short time periods of preoperative warming in the prevention of perioperative hypothermia. Anaesthesia 2012;67:612–7.

35. Sessler DI, Schroeder M, Merrifield B, et al. Optimal duration and temperature of pre-warming. Anesthesiology 1995;82:674–81.

36. Leslie K, Sessler DI. Perioperative hypothermia in the high-risk surgical patient. Best Pract Res Clin Anaesthesiol 2003;17(4):485–98.

37. Leben J, Tryba M. Prevention of hypothermia during surgery: contribution of convective heating system and warm infusion. Ann N Y Acad Sci 1997;813:807–11.

38. Robles-Cervantes JA, Martinez-Molina R, Cardenas-Camarena L. Heating infiltration solutions used in tumescent liposuction: minimizing surgical risk. Plast Reconstr Surg 2005;116:1077–81.

39. Hirshey Dirksen SJ, Larach MG, Rosenberg H, et al. Future directions in malignant hyperthermia research and patient care. Anesth Analg 2011;113:1108–19.

40. Halsall PJ, Cain PA, Ellis FR. Retrospective analysis of anaesthetics received by patients before susceptibility to malignant hyperpyrexia was recognized. Br J Anaesth 1979;51:949–54.

41. Brady JE, Sun LS, Rosenberg H, et al. Prevalence of malignant hyperthermia due to anesthesia in New York State, 2001-2005. Anesth Analg 2009;109:1162–6.

42. Available at: http://www.aboutlawsuits.com/anesthesia-malpractice-lawsuit-malignant-hyperthermia-death-6174/. Accessed October 9, 2012.

43. The guidelines are available at: http://www.aaaasf.org/pub/htm. Accessed October 9, 2012.

44. Larach MG, Gronert GA, Allen GC, et al. Clinical presentation, treatment, and complications of malignant hyperthermia in North America from 1987 to 2006. Anesth Analg 2010;110:498–507.

45. Kobayashi S, Bannister ML, Gagopadhyay J, et al. Dantrolene stabilizes domain interactions within the ryanodine receptor. J Biol Chem 2005;280:6580–7.

46. Larach MG, Hirshey Dirksen SJ, Belani KG, et al. Creation of a guide for the transfer of the malignant hyperthermia patient from ambulatory surgery centers to receiving hospital facilities. Anesth Analg 2012;114(1):94–100.

47. Annadata RS, Sessler DI, Tayefeh F, et al. Desflurane slightly increases the sweating threshold, but produces marked, non-linear decreases in the vasoconstriction and shivering thresholds. Anesthesiology 1995;83:1205–11.

48. Talke P, Tayefeh F, Sessler DI, et al. Dexmedetomidine does not alter the sweating threshold, but comparably and linearly reduces the vasoconstriction and shivering thresholds. Anesthesiology 1997;87:835–41.

Infections in Outpatient Surgery

Sheila S. Nazarian Mobin, MD, MMM[a],
Geoffrey R. Keyes, MD[*,b], Robert Singer, MD[c],
James Yates, MD[d,e,f,g,h], Dennis Thompson, MD, FACS[i]

KEYWORDS

- Outpatient surgery • Infections • Plastic surgery • Postoperative care

KEY POINTS

- In the plastic surgery patient population, outpatient surgery is cost effective and will continue to grow as the preferred arena for performing surgery in healthy patients.
- Although there is a widespread myth that outpatient surgery centers may suffer from increased infection rates due to lax infection control, the data presented from American Association for Accreditation of Ambulatory Surgery Facilities (AAAASF)–accredited facilities prove the contrary.
- There is a lack of data investigating infection prevention in the perioperative period in plastic surgery patients.
- As data collection becomes more refined, tracking the postoperative care environment should offer additional opportunities to lower the incidence of postoperative infections.

INTRODUCTION

Over the last decade, surgical care in the United States has shifted to an ambulatory surgical setting, where enormous growth has been seen. Ambulatory surgical centers are defined by the Centers for Medicare & Medicaid Services as facilities that operate exclusively to provide surgical services to patients who do not require hospitalization or stays in a surgical facility longer than 24 hours.[1] Between 2001 and 2008, there was a greater than 50% increase in the number of Medicare-certified ambulatory surgical centers in the United States.[2,3] In 2007, these facilities performed more than 6 million procedures.[2] According to Reuters,[4] as of 2011, more than 57 million outpatient surgeries took place in the United States in more than 5000 surgery centers nationwide. With efforts to boost cost-savings, three-quarters of surgeries are done on an outpatient basis.[5]

With growth in this sector, there have been articles written that express concern about the level of infection control in the outpatient surgery environment. These concerns have been fueled by some high-profile examples of lapses in prevention. Between 1998 and 2008, 448 people acquired hepatitis B or hepatitis C infection linked to outpatient care in 33 outbreaks.[5] In a 2010 *JAMA* article,[5] an audit of 68 centers in 3 states participating in a pilot inspection program found that approximately two-thirds (67.6%) had a lapse in at least 1 of 5 infection control categories. Although only a pilot study, these findings set off concerns about

[a] Resident Physician, Division of Plastic Surgery, Keck School of Medicine of USC, 1510 San Pablo Street, Suite 415, Los Angeles, CA 90033, USA; [b] Department of Plastic Surgery, Keck School of Medicine, University of Southern California, Los Angeles, CA, USA; [c] American Society of Plastic Surgeons, La Jolla, CA, USA; [d] Plastic and Cosmetic Surgery Center, Camp Hill, Pennsylvania, USA; [e] Grandview Surgery and Laser Center, Camp Hill, Pennsylvania, USA; [f] Holy Spirit Hospital, Camp Hill, Pennsylvania, USA; [g] Plastic Surgery Department, Pinnacle Health System, Harrisburg, Pennsylvania, USA; [h] AAAASF, Gurnee, Illinois, USA; [i] Department of Plastic Surgery, University of California, Los Angeles, CA, USA
* Corresponding author.
E-mail address: geoffreykeyes@sbcglobal.net

Clin Plastic Surg 40 (2013) 439–446
http://dx.doi.org/10.1016/j.cps.2013.04.009
0094-1298/13/$ – see front matter © 2013 Elsevier Inc. All rights reserved.

Table 1
The total number of untoward operative sequelae

Total cases all AAAASF specialties	5,416,071		
Total procedures all AAAASF specialties	7,629,686	1.41	Procedures per case
Plastic surgery cases	3,922,202		
Plastic surgery procedures	5,525,255	1.41	Procedures per case

potentially serious lapses in infection control in several states.

The Centers for Disease Control and Prevention assess 5 categories of infection control: hand hygiene and personal protective equipment, injection safety and medication handling, equipment reprocessing (eg, sterilization and high-level disinfection), environmental cleaning, and handling of blood glucose monitoring equipment. The Centers for Disease Control and Prevention have found errors in basic infection control practices in the outpatient setting and, as a result, the reputation of outpatient surgery centers has suffered. More recent findings, however, in an extensive review of the data collection from the AAAASF, suggest that outpatient surgeries performed in accredited centers have low infection rates.[6]

DATA ON INFECTION RATES IN OUTPATIENT SURGERY FROM AAAASF

Data collected from AAAASF-certified surgery centers from 2001 to 2012 (**Table 1**) analyzed outcomes from 5,416,071 operations, where 7,629,686 procedures were performed (1.41 procedures per case). Plastic surgery cases comprised 3,922,202 of these operations and 5,525,255 of the procedures (also, 1.41 procedures per case).

The total number of untoward operative sequelae from these 3,922,202 plastic surgery cases was 21,944 (0.4052%); that is, 1 in 247 plastic surgery cases or 1 in 348 plastic surgery procedures had a complication (**Table 2**). Of these complications, 3063 were infections (0.0781%). Infections developed in 1 in 1281 plastic surgery cases and 1 in 1804 plastic surgery procedures. The infection rate as a percentage of all untoward sequelae was 13.96%.

In this data set, infection was most commonly reported, in order from highest to lowest, in the following procedures: breast augmentation, abdominoplasty, breast lift/reduction, liposuction, and facelift (**Table 3**). Although more infections were reported with breast augmentation surgery, there were more breast augmentations performed and the rate of infection was lower than in patients undergoing abdominoplasty. Therefore, the rate of infection per procedure, from highest to lowest, was as follows: abdominoplasty, breast lift/reduction, breast augmentation, liposuction, and facelift.

A total 462,588 abdominoplasties were performed and 757 cases of infection reported. This is a 0.16% infection rate (1 in 611 patients) from abdominoplasty. Also, 1,125,274 breast augmentation procedures were evaluated and 921 infections reported, resulting in a 0.08% incidence of infection or 1 in 1222 patients; 515,252 patients underwent breast lift/reduction with 582 reported infections, which is a 0.11% infection rate, or 1 in 885 breast lift/reduction patients; 517 of 688,241 liposuction patients had reported infection— 0.08% or 1 in 1331 liposuction patients; and 346 of 499,477 facelift patients developed infection— 0.07% or 1 in 1444 facelift patients (see **Table 3**). The most commonly cultured organism was Staphylococcus (**Table 4**). No organisms were found or

Table 2
Incidence of infection[a]

		Incidence Percentage by Case	1 in # Case	Incidence Percentage by Procedure	1 in # Procedure
Total plastic surgery sequelae	21,944	0.41%	247	0.29%	348
Total plastic surgery infections	3063	0.08%	1281	0.06%	1804
Infections as percentage of sequelae	13.96%				

[a] Incidence of infection by case and procedure. Infection as a percentage of all plastic surgery sequelae.

Table 3
Five procedures most commonly associated with infection

Procedure	Number of Infections	Number of Cases	Rate of Infection (%)	1 in
Breast augmentation	921	1,125,274	0.08	1222
Abdominoplasty	757	462,588	0.16	611
Breast lift/reduction	582	515,252	0.11	885
Liposuction	517	688,241	0.08	1331
Facelift and related procedures	346	499,477	0.07	1444

no culture was taken in 420 cases. Methicillin-resistant *Staphylococcus aureus* (MRSA) was cultured in 86 cases.

A total 225 plastic surgery patients had to be hospitalized due to postoperative infection. Most commonly, these patients requiring hospitalization had undergone, in order of most common to least common: abdominoplasty, breast augmentation, liposuction, breast lift/reduction, and facelift (**Table 5**). The specific incidences of infection requiring hospitalization from each plastic surgery procedure are as follows: 1 in 5782 abdominoplasty patients; 1 in 32,151 breast augmentation patients; 1 in 36,804 breast lift/reduction patients; 1 in 45,883 liposuction patients; and 1 in 49,948 facelift patients (see **Table 5**). The most commonly found organism in these patients was also Staphylococcus (**Table 6**). Cultures were not performed in 20 cases and cultures were negative in 12. MRSA was present in 9 patients requiring hospitalization because of infection.

Among these patients who acquired infections after plastic surgical procedures, only 1 succumbed. This patient had undergone liposuction and developed a MRSA infection. Thus, the incidence of mortality from all plastic surgery infections performed in an outpatient setting is 0.03%, or 1 death in 3063 infections. The death rate from infection among all plastic surgery cases performed in an outpatient setting is 0.00003%, or 1 death in 3,922,202 cases.

Table 4
Most common organisms

Organism	Number of Cases
Staphylococcus	376
Culture not done	240
No growth	180
MRSA	86

COMPARING INFECTION RATES BETWEEN INPATIENT AND OUTPATIENT SURGERIES

Comparing infection rates in hospital-based operations to outpatient facilities may seem an exercise in futility. Operations performed in hospitals may be performed on patients with higher levels of comorbidity and anesthetic risk than performed on an outpatient basis. Comparing specific procedures in similar patients, however, in the 2 settings is useful.

Speigleman and colleagues[7] performed a retrospective study on 69 consecutive abdominoplasties: 37 inpatients and 32 outpatients. Although the inpatients were on average older and had higher body mass indices, these differences did not reach statistical significance. The weight of the pannus removed from inpatients was significantly higher and this can be explained by the higher body mass indices in this group. The operations took longer in the inpatient group, although not significantly. The investigators defined wound infection as any patient who started on cloxacillin due to erythema or cellulitis near the surgical wound. Only 1 of 32 outpatients had a postoperative infection (3.1%), whereas 4 of 37 inpatients had postoperative infections (10.8%). On average, inpatients incurred an extra $1500 for the first night of hospital stay and $1000 for the second night. The outpatient group avoided these costs. The investigators strongly endorsed the safety and efficacy of abdominoplasties performed in an outpatient setting with a clear cost benefit.

In another study, by Buenaventura and colleagues[8] breast reductions performed in either setting were examined over a 3-year period. Of the patients examined, 286 were outpatients and 52 were inpatients. The inpatients were, on average, 8 years older and 8 kg heavier and had approximately 400 g more breast tissue resected than the outpatients undergoing reduction mammoplasty. There were no significant differences in the incidence of minor complications, including infections, and the investigators concluded that

Table 5
Hospitalizations from infection

Procedure	Number of Hospitalizations	Number of Cases	Rate of Infection	1 in
Abdominoplasty	80	462,588	0.0173%	5782
Breast augmentation	35	1,125,274	0.0031%	32,151
Liposuction	15	688,241	0.0022%	45,883
Breast lift/reduction	14	515,252	0.0027%	36,804
Facelift and related procedures	10	499,477	0.0020%	49,948
Total	225			

reduction mammoplasty could be performed safely in an outpatient setting, with an average cost savings of between $1500 and $2500 compared with an overnight stay.

A retrospective study performed by Byrd and colleagues[9] reviewed 5316 consecutive cases performed in an outpatient setting between 1995 and 2000. Most cases were aesthetic in nature. Complications requiring a return to an operating room were analyzed, as were infection rates. They found that during this 6-year-period, 35 complications and no deaths were reported; 77% of complications were hematomas. There were only 6 infections reported. Infections requiring a return to an operating room accounted for only 0.11% of patients. Furthermore, 10.2% of cases performed consisted of a combination of multiple plastic surgery procedures. No greater risk of infection or increased adverse outcome was attributed to performing more than 1 procedure during a case in this study.

PATIENT SELECTION TO REDUCE INFECTION RATES

With the clear cost savings in avoiding inpatient stays, there is incentive to performing safe outpatient surgeries to keep this option viable. There are evidence-based precautions to take to keep outpatient infection rates low. Careful patient selection is the first step. Smoking, alcohol abuse, poor blood sugar control, obesity (greater than 20% of ideal body weight), steroid use, and malnutrition can all lead to poor wound healing and infection of open wounds.

Smoking

In an effort to clarify how smoking and nicotine affect wound healing, Sorensen[10] performed a review in 2012 and ultimately included 177 articles. He found that smoking decreases tissue oxygenation and attenuates the inflammatory healing process by way of cell chemotactic responsiveness, migratory function, and oxidative bactericidal mechanisms. The proliferative response is impaired by a reduced fibroblast migration and proliferations and decreased collagen synthesis and deposition. Smoking cessation restores tissue oxygenation and metabolism rapidly. Inflammatory cell response is reversed, in part, within 4 weeks, whereas the proliferative response remains impaired. Nicotine does not affect tissue microenvironment but seems to impair inflammation and stimulate proliferation. Cotinine or nicotine may be ordered as a blood or urine test to evaluate compliance.

Alcohol Use

Tonnensen and Kehlet[11] performed a meta-analysis to identify articles published from 1967 to 1998 looking at postoperative morbidity in alcohol abusers (more than 5 drinks of 60-g ethanol per day for several months or years). Studies demonstrated a 2-fold to 3-fold increase in postoperative morbidity; the most frequent complications were infections, bleeding, and cardiopulmonary insufficiency. Wound complications contributed to half of the morbidity. This study reported that the risk of wound complications is probably due to a combination of suppressed immune function, impaired hemostasis, and reduced

Table 6
Most common organisms in hospitalized patients

Bacteria	Number of Cases
Staphylococcus	35
Culture not done	20
No growth	12
MRSA	9

wound healing. According to Jorgensen and colleagues[12,13] in 2 separate studies, there is a reduced amount of protein and collagen in wounds in alcohol users that improves with 8 weeks of abstinence.

Poor Blood Glucose Control

Maintaining normal blood glucose levels has also been shown to lower the risk of infection. Hyperglycemia is associated with impaired leukocyte function, including granulocyte adherence, impaired phagocytosis, delayed chemotaxis, and depressed bactericidal capacity.[14] These leukocyte deficiencies can lead to infection and improve with tight glycemic control; however, the optimal targeted blood glucose to reduce postoperative infections is not known.

Obesity

Wick and colleagues[15] performed a retrospective cohort study of 7020 colectomy patients using claims from insurance plans. Patients who had a total or segmental colectomy over 6 years were included. They compared 30-day surgical site infection (SSI) rates among obese and nonobese patients and statistical analysis was performed to identify risk factors for SSIs. They found that obese patients had an increased rate of SSIs compared with nonobese patients (14.5% vs 9.5%, respectively; $P<.001$). The mean total cost was $31,933 in patients with infection versus $14,608 in patients without infection ($P<.001$). Total length of stay was longer in patients with infection than in those without infection (mean, 9.5 vs 8.1 days, respectively; $P<.001$), as was the probability of hospital readmission (27.8% vs 6.8%, respectively; $P<.001$). They concluded that obesity increases the risk of an SSI after colectomy by 60%, and the presence of infection increases the colectomy cost by a mean of $17,324.

Steroid use

A study by Ismael and colleagues[16] looked at preoperative steroid use and its association with increased postoperative complications. They used the National Surgical Quality Improvement Program public use files from 2005 to 2008 and found that of 635,265 patients identified, 20,434 (3.2%) used steroids preoperatively. Superficial SSIs increased from 2.9% to 5% of those patients using steroids (odds ratio [OR] 1.724). Deep SSIs increased from 0.8% to 1.8% (OR 2.353). Organ/space SSIs and dehiscence increased 2-fold to 3-fold with steroid use (ORs 2.469 and 3.338, respectively). Mortality increased almost 4-fold (1.6%–6.0%; OR 3.920). All results were significant ($P<.001$). The investigators concluded that

concerns related to surgical risks in patients on chronic steroid regimens seem valid.

Malnutrition

It is generally thought that severe protein malnutrition may lead to poor wound healing and, therefore, a higher risk of SSIs. In a study by Markel and colleagues,[17] pediatric patients with ulcerative colitis were included in a 10-year retrospective review. A total of 51 children were identified and 20 infectious complications were identified in 18 patients. Preoperative steroid use was associated with a greater postoperative wound infection rate. Preoperative hemoglobin less than 10 g/dL ($P<.05$) and albumin less than 3 g/dL ($P = .1$) were associated with greater rates of postoperative infection.

To evaluate the impact of nutritional support on clinical outcomes in patients at nutritional risk defined by the nutritional risk screening 2002, Jie and colleagues[18] performed a prospective cohort study of hospitalized patients from 3 departments at The Johns Hopkins Hospital in Baltimore and 2 teaching hospitals in Beijing, from March 2007 to May 2008. Data were collected on the nutritional risk screening, application for parenteral nutrition and enteral nutrition, surgery, complications, and length of stay. The investigators recruited 1831 patients, with 45.2% of them at nutritional risk. Among the at-risk patients, the complication rate was significantly lower in the nutritional-support group than in the no-support group (20.3% vs 28.1%, $P = .009$), mainly because of the lower rate of infectious complications (10.5% vs 18.9%, $P<.001$). Subgroup analysis showed the complication rate was significantly lower in the enteral nutrition group ($P<.001$) but not the parenteral nutrition group ($P = .29$) compared with the no-support group. Among the patients without nutritional risk, the complication rate was not different between the nutritional-support group and the no-support group ($P = .10$). Statistical analysis showed nutritional support was a protective factor for complications in at-risk patients when adjusted for confounders ($P<.001$). No difference in length of stay was found.

Preoperative and Perioperative Methods to Reduce Surgical Site Infections

Perioperative antibiotics

The Centers for Medicare & Medicaid Services, in the form of the Surgical Care Improvement Project, have mandated prophylactic, preoperative, and perioperative antibiotic use. This evidence-based initiative targeted a 25% reduction in elective surgical complications, such as SSIs, by 2010.[19] A cornerstone of the Surgical Care Improvement Project guidelines focused on SSI prevention is not only the provision of prophylactic antibiotics but also the administration of the appropriate prophylactic antibiotic within 1 hour before elective surgical incisions and cessation of the antibiotic within 24 hours of surgery.[20]

Although there have been recommendations to limit the use of perioperative prophylactic antibiotics, there are not many studies reported for plastic surgery patients. A study by Clayton and colleagues,[21] instituted antibiotic prescribing guidelines based on the Surgical Care Improvement Project. An increased rate of SSIs, similar to AAAASF data, was noted in breast reconstruction patients. The investigators sought to determine whether the change in antibiotic prophylaxis regimen affected rates of SSIs. They performed a retrospective study comparing patients undergoing breast reconstruction who received preoperative and postoperative prophylactic antibiotics with a group who received only a single dose of preoperative antibiotic. The type of reconstruction and known risk factors for implant infection were noted and 250 patients were included: 116 in the presurgical care improvement project group received preoperative and postoperative prophylactic antibiotics, and 134 in the surgical care improvement project group received a single dose of preoperative antibiotic. The overall rate of SSIs increased from 18.1% to 34.3% ($P = .004$) in those receiving the single dose of preoperative antibiotic. Infections requiring reoperation increased from 4.3% to 16.4% ($P = .002$). Multivariate logistic regression demonstrated that patients in the surgical care improvement group were 4.74 times more likely to develop an SSI requiring reoperation (95% CI, 1.69–13.80). Obesity, history of radiation therapy, and reconstruction with tissue expanders were associated with increased rates of SSI requiring reoperation. The investigators concluded that withholding postoperative prophylactic antibiotics in prosthetic breast reconstruction is associated with an increased risk of SSI, reoperation, and thus reconstructive failure. They suggested further studies to delineate the optimal amount of time to continue postoperative antibiotics.

Antibiotic saline irrigation

A study by Pfeiffer and colleagues[22] included 436 women who underwent breast augmentation at 2 different times by a single surgeon. The first group underwent surgery with cephalothin added to the saline irrigation; the second group was irrigated with saline alone—99.8% of patients underwent subpectoral placement with periareolar incisions. The frequency of infection in the cephalothin group was much less (6.7% vs 12.8% in the normal saline-only group, $P = .044$). The frequency of seroma was also less in the cephalothin group (7.6% vs 2.9%, $P = .036$). There was no significant difference in the development of capsular contraction between the 2 groups.

Intranasal mupirocin

A 2008 study by van Rijen and colleagues[23] showed that the prophylactic use of intranasal mupirocin significantly reduced the rate of postoperative *Staphylococcus aureus* infections among carriers. It has been shown that a large proportion of *S aureus* infections originate from patients' own flora.[24–26] Approximately 30% of the population carries nasal *S aureus* and present a risk factor for subsequent infection in patients undergoing surgery.[27–29] A literature search was performed and 686 surgical patients treated with 2% mupirocin calcium ointment, a broad-spectrum topical antibiotic, were reviewed. There were fewer *S aureus* infections found with treatment, 25 (3.6%) compared with 46 (6.7%) in the controls. This was a significant decrease in the incidence of *S aureus* nosocomial infection among surgical patients. Cases of mupirocin resistant *S aureus* have been reported in some patients with repeated use.[30]

Normothermia

Keeping the temperature of the patient above 35°C has also been shown to have an effect on decreasing SSIs. In a study by Seamon and colleagues,[31] 524 trauma laparotomies were analyzed from 2003 to 2008. The mean operative nadir temperature of the study population was 35.2 ± 1.1°C and 30.5% had at least 1 temperature measurement less than 35°C. Patients who developed SSIs (36.1%) had a lower mean intraoperative temperature nadir ($P = .009$) and had a greater number of intraoperative temperature measurements less than 35°C ($P<.001$) than those who did not. Statistical analysis showed that an intraoperative temperature of 35°C as the nadir temperature most predictive of SSI development. Multivariate analysis determined that a single intraoperative temperature measurement less than 35°C independently increased the site infection risk 221% per degree below 35°C ($P = .007$).

Preoperative hair removal

Although preparation of people for surgery has traditionally included removal of hair from the incision site, some studies claim that preoperative hair removal is harmful and causes SSIs and should be avoided. Tanner and colleagues[32] performed a Cochrane Database review to determine if routine preoperative hair removal (compared with no removal) and if the timing or method of hair removal influenced rates of SSIs. Fourteen trials (17 comparisons) were included in the review; 3 trials involved multiple comparisons. Six trials, 2 of which had 3 comparison arms (972 participants), compared hair removal (shaving, clipping, or depilatory cream) with no hair removal and found no statistically significant difference in SSI rates; however, the comparison was underpowered. Three trials (1343 participants) that compared shaving with clipping showed significantly more SSIs associated with shaving (relative risk [RR] 2.09; 95% CI, 1.15–3.80). Seven trials (1213 participants) found no significant difference in SSI rates when hair removal by shaving was compared with depilatory cream (RR 1.53; 95% CI, 0.73–3.21); however, this comparison was also underpowered. One trial compared 2 groups that shaved or clipped hair on the day of surgery compared with the day before surgery. There was no statistically significant difference in the number of SSIs between groups; however, this comparison was also underpowered. The study investigators identified no trials that compared clipping with depilatory cream, investigated application of depilatory cream at different preoperative time points, or investigated hair removal in different settings (eg, ward or preoperative holding area). They concluded that when it is necessary to remove hair, the existing evidence suggests that clippers are associated with fewer SSIs than razors. There was no significant difference in SSI rates between depilatory creams and shaving or between shaving or clipping the day before surgery or on the day of surgery; however, studies were small and more research is needed.

Chlorhexadine shower

Chlorhexidine showering is frequently recommended as an important preoperative measure to prevent SSIs. The efficacy of this approach was evaluated by Chlebicki and colleagues.[33] They performed a search of electronic databases to identify prospective controlled trials evaluating whole-body preoperative bathing with chlorhexidine versus placebo or no bath for prevention of SSIs. Sixteen trials met inclusion criteria with a total of 17,932 patients: 7952 patients received a chlorhexidine bath, and 9980 patients were allocated to comparator groups. Overall, 6.8% of patients developed SSIs in the chlorhexidine group compared with 7.2% of patients in the comparator groups. Chlorhexidine bathing did not significantly reduce overall incidence of SSIs when compared with soap, placebo, or no shower or bath (RR 0.90; 95% CI, 0.77–1.05; $P = .19$). The investigators concluded that the available clinical trials suggest no appreciable benefit of preoperative whole-body chlorhexidine bathing for prevention of SSIs.

SUMMARY

In the plastic surgery patient population, outpatient surgery is cost effective and will continue to grow as the preferred arena for performing surgery in healthy patients. Although there is a widespread myth that outpatient surgery centers may suffer from increased infection rates due to lax infection control, the data presented from AAAASF accredited facilities prove the contrary.

There is a lack of data investigating infection prevention in the perioperative period in plastic surgery patients. Therefore, much of the data discussed in this article is extrapolated from literature in other surgical specialties, such as colorectal, trauma, orthopedic, and cardiothoracic surgery. As data collection becomes more refined, tracking the postoperative care environment should offer additional opportunities to lower the incidence of postoperative infections.

REFERENCES

1. Medicare program: changes to the ambulatory surgical center payment system and CY 2009 payment rates: final rule. Fed Regist 2008;73(223):68714.
2. Healthcare-associated infections: HHS action needed to obtain nationally representative data on risk in ambulatory surgical centers. GAO-09-213, February 25, 2009. US Government Accountability Office. Available at: http://nueterrahealthcare.com/building_partnerships/documents/GAOHAlreport 02-09.pdf. Accessed May 10, 2010.
3. A data book: healthcare spending and the medicare program. Medicare Payment Advisory Commission (MedPAC); 2009. Available at: http://www.medpac.gov/documents/Jun09DataBookEntireReport.pdf. Accessed October 31, 2009.
4. McCook A. More outpatient surgery centers, more surgeries. 2011. Available at: http://www.reuters.com/article/2011/02/23/us-outpatient-surgery-idUS TRE71M4XQ20110223. Accessed Feb 23, 2011.
5. Schaefer MK, Jhung M, Dahl M, et al. Infection control assessment of ambulatory surgical centers. JAMA 2010;303(22):2273–9.
6. Keyes GR, Singer R, Iverson RE, et al. Analysis of outpatient surgery center safety using an internet-based quality improvement and peer review program. Plast Reconstr Surg 2004;113(6):1760–70.
7. Spiegelman JI, Levine RH. Abdominoplasty: a comparison of outpatient and inpatient procedures shows that it is a safe and effective procedure for outpatients in an office-based surgery clinic. Plast Reconstr Surg 2006;118(2):517–22.

8. Buenaventura S, Severinac R, Mullis W, et al. Outpatient reduction mammaplasty: a review of 338 consecutive cases. Ann Plast Surg 1996;36(2):162–6.

9. Byrd HS, Barton FE, Orenstein HH, et al. Safety and efficacy in an accredited outpatient plastic surgery facility: a review of 5316 cases. Plast Reconstr Surg 2003;112(2):636–41.

10. Sorensen LT. Wound healing and infection in surgery: the pathophysiological impact of smoking, smoking cessation, and nicotine replacement therapy. A systematic review. Ann Surg 2012;255(6):1069–79.

11. Tonnesen H, Kehlet H. Preoperative alcoholism and postoperative morbidity. Br J Surg 1999;86: 869–74.

12. Jorgensen LN, Tonnesen H, Pedersen S, et al. Reduced amounts of total protein in artificial wounds of alcohol abusers. Br J Surg 1998;85(Suppl 2):152–3.

13. Jorgensen LN, Kallehave F, Karlsmark T, et al. Reduced collagen accumulation after major surgery. Br J Surg 1996;83:1591–4.

14. Latham R, Lancaster AD, Covington JF, et al. The association of diabetes and glucose control with surgical site infections among cardiothoracic surgery patients. Infect Control Hosp Epidemiol 2001;22: 607–12.

15. Wick EC, Hirose K, Clark JM, et al. Surgical site infections and cost in obese patients undergoing colorectal surgery. Arch Surg 2011;146(9):1068–72.

16. Ismael H, Horst M, Farooq M, et al. Adverse effects of preoperative steroid use on surgical outcomes. Am J Surg 2011;201(3):305–8.

17. Markel TA, Lou DC, Pfefferkorn M, et al. Steroids and poor nutrition are associated with infectious wound complications in children undergoing first stage procedures for ulcerative colitis. Surgery 2008;144(4): 540–5.

18. Jie B, Jiang ZM, Nolan MT, et al. Impact of nutritional support on clinical outcome in patients at nutritional risk: a multicenter, prospective cohort study in Baltimore and Beijing teaching hospitals. Nutrition 2010; 26(11–12):1088–93.

19. Griffin FA. Reducing surgical complications: five million lives campaign. Jt Comm J Qual Patient Saf 2007;33:660–5.

20. Berenguer CM, Ochsner MG, Lord SA, et al. Improving surgical site infections: using National Surgical Quality Improvement Program data to institute Surgical Care Improvement Project protocols in improving surgical outcomes. J Am Coll Surg 2010; 210:737–43.

21. Clayton JL, Bazakas A, Lee CN, et al. Once is not enough: withholding postoperative prophylactic antibiotics in prosthetic breast reconstruction is associated with an increased risk of infection. Plast Reconstr Surg 2012;130(3):495–502.

22. Pfeiffer P, Jorgensen S, Kristiansen TB, et al. Protective effect of topical antibiotics in breast augmentation. Plast Reconstr Surg 2009;124:629.

23. Van Rijen MM, Bonten M, Wenzel RP, et al. Intranasal mupirocin for reduction of Staphylococcus aureus infections in surgical patients with nasal carriage: a systematic review. J Antimicrob Chemother 2008; 61(2):254–61.

24. Von Eiff C, Becker K, Machka K, et al. Nasal carriage as a source of taphylococcus aureus bacteremia. Sutdy Group. N Engl J Med 2001;344:11–6.

25. Wertheim HF, Vos MC, Ott A, et al. Risk and outcome of nosocomial Staphylococcus aureus bacteraemia in nasal carriers versus non-carriers. Lancet 2004; 364:703–5.

26. Kluytmans JA, Mouton JW, Ijzerman EP, et al. Nasal carriage of S. aureus as a major risk factor for wound infections after cardiac surgery. J Infect Dis 1995; 171:216–9.

27. Kalmeijer MD, Van Nieuwland-Bollen E, Bogaers-Hofman D, et al. Nasal carriage of Staphylococcus aureus is a major risk factor for surgical-site infections in orthopedic surgery. Infect Control Hosp Epidemiol 2000;21:319–23.

28. Kluytmans J, van Belkum A, Verbrugh H. Nasal carriage of Staphylococcus aureus: epidemiology, underlying mechanisms, and associated risks. Clin Microbiol Rev 1997;10:505–20.

29. Mangram AJ, Horan TC, Pearson ML, et al. The hospital infection control practices advisory committee guideline for prevention of surgical site infection. Infect Control Hosp Epidemiol 1999;20:250–78.

30. Jones JC, Rogers TJ, Brookmeyer P, et al. Mupirocin resistance in patients colonized with methicillin resistant staphylococcus aureus in a surgical intensive care unit. Clin Infect Dis 2007;45:541–7.

31. Seamon MJ, Wobb J, Gaughan JP, et al. The effects of intraoperative hypothermia on surgical site infection: an analysis of 524 trauma laparotomies. Ann Surg 2012;255(4):789–95.

32. Tanner J, Norrie P, Melen K. Preoperative hair removal to reduce surgical site infection. Update of Cochrane Database Syst Rev 2006;(3):CD004122. Cochrane Database of Systematic Reviews. (11): CD004122, 2011.

33. Chlebicki MP, Safdar N, O'Horo JC, et al. Preoperative chlorhexidine shower or bath for prevention of surgical site infection: a meta-analysis. Am J Infect Control 2013;41(2):167–73.

Management of Postoperative Nausea and Vomiting in Ambulatory Surgery
The Big Little Problem

Mary Keyes, MD

KEYWORDS

- Postoperative nausea and vomiting • PONV prophylaxis • PONV in ambulatory surgery

KEY POINTS

- The Consensus Guidelines for Managing Postoperative Nausea and Vomiting (PONV) provides an evidence-based management strategy for clinicians.
- Although the exact cause of PONV is unknown, many receptors, pathways, and neurotransmitters are likely involved. Because of the multitude of inputs that may be causal, single therapies are often inadequate.
- An individual's risk for PONV is best predicted by using a simplified risk score of independent predictors: female gender, nonsmoking status, history of PONV or motion sickness, and postoperative opioid use.
- Although some types of surgery, plastic surgery among them, are associated with higher PONV risk, risk scores that include type of surgery provide no greater predictive value.
- Strategies that avoid inhaled anesthetics such as total intravenous anesthesia (TIVA), elimination of nitrous oxide, and minimal opioid use reduce risk.
- Multimodal regimens involving TIVA with propofol, combination antiemetic prophylaxis, hydration, and nonnarcotic analgesics, are the most effective way to prevent PONV in high-risk patients.
- Postdischarge nausea and vomiting is common in ambulatory surgery patients. Those who have nausea in the postanesthesia care unit (PACU) are particularly at risk. Which agents in addition to dexamethasone are effective remains to be determined.

Considerable progress has been made in the management of postoperative nausea and vomiting (PONV) since it was labeled the big little problem over 20 years ago by Kapur.[1] Although usually self-limited, it is distressing to patients who, in some studies, state they would pay up to $100.00 out of pocket for a drug to avoid it.[2] PONV can lead to dehydration, electrolyte disturbances, and the inability to take vital oral medications and fluids after surgery. The act of vomiting can cause suture disruption, lead to hematoma formation, and be a risk factor for pulmonary aspiration. Its occurrence often delays discharge from ambulatory settings and is a leading cause of unanticipated hospital admission escalating health care costs. With most surgeries now being done on an outpatient or ambulatory basis, considerable attention is being given to this issue.

The Consensus Guidelines for Managing Postoperative Nausea and Vomiting authored by an international panel of experts created an evidence-based management strategy for clinicians.[3] These

UCLA Department of Anesthesiology, Ronald Reagan UCLA Medical Center, 757 Westwood Plaza, Suite 3325, Los Angeles, CA 90095-7403, USA
E-mail address: mkeyes@mednet.ucla.edu

Clin Plastic Surg 40 (2013) 447–452
http://dx.doi.org/10.1016/j.cps.2013.04.007
0094-1298/13/$ – see front matter Published by Elsevier Inc.

guidelines have been the foundation for the improved understanding and recent advances gained regarding this common, undesirable perioperative experience. However, there is still room for improvement, particularly in the area of postdischarge nausea and vomiting (PDNV), which occurred in up to 37% of ambulatory patients in a recently published study.[4]

PATHOPHYSIOLOGY OF NAUSEA AND VOMITING

Various stimuli that produce nausea and vomiting converge in an area of the medulla known as the emetic center. This center is not a discrete nucleus but rather a collection of neurons controlled by a central pattern generator. Input to the emetic center comes from a variety of pathways: the visceral afferent nerves of the gastrointestinal tract, the chemoreceptor trigger zone (CTZ), the cerebral cortex, and the vestibular apparatus. Each of these systems is modulated by specific receptors and neurotransmitters. The CTZ is located in the fourth ventricle of the brainstem but, because of its uniquely permeable membrane, it is outside the blood-brain barrier, which allows detection of toxins and drugs in the circulation. Stimulation of dopamine, opioid, histamine, acetylcholine, serotonin type 3 receptors, or neurokinin-1 receptors in the emetic center initiates the vomiting reflex. Therapies that interfere with each of these neurotransmitter-receptor interactions are used to prevent nausea and vomiting in clinical practice. Because of the multitude of inputs that may be causal in the production of nausea and vomiting, single therapies are often inadequate.

ASSESSING RISK FOR PONV

The important first step in managing PONV is to assess risk for each patient. In doing so, there are 3 categories of factors to consider:

Patient-specific factors:

1. Female gender
2. Nonsmoking status
3. History of PONV or motion sickness

Anesthesia-related factors:

1. Use of volatile anesthetics
2. Use of nitrous oxide
3. Perioperative opioid use

Surgery-related factors:

1. Duration and invasiveness of surgery
2. Type of surgery

A simplified risk score of independent predictors by Apfel and colleagues[5] has gained widespread recognition and implementation by anesthesia providers. Although some types of surgery (plastic, strabismus, gynecologic, laparoscopic, urologic) are known to be associated with a higher PONV risk, risk scores that include type of surgery provide no greater predictive value than a simplified version. For example, hysterectomy is known to have a higher PONV risk. It may be that this increased risk is a reflection of the patient population who are female (the strongest risk factor) rather than the surgery itself. Patients having plastic surgery are predominantly women, making them inherently at higher risk. The simplified risk score for an adult having a balanced inhalational anesthetic consists of the following 4 factors: female gender, nonsmoking status, previous history of PONV or motion sickness, and postoperative opioid use. The presence of 1 risk factor correlates with a risk of 20% for PONV. Each additional risk factor adds 20%, so that patients with all 4 have an 80% risk of developing PONV (**Fig. 1**).

REDUCING RISK

There are often strategies that can be incorporated into the anesthesia and surgical plan to reduce the probability of developing PONV:

1. Total intravenous anesthesia (TIVA) with propofol reduces PONV risk about 19% from a patient's baseline risk.[6] Impediments to the use of propofol have been cost, the lack of ability to monitor depth of anesthesia, and the need for an infusion pump. Propofol is now a generic drug, making the cost difference between it and a volatile agent much less significant. The cost savings gained in having less PONV and improved patient satisfaction may justify the increased cost.
2. Nitrous oxide use is a risk factor for PONV, although not as significant as the volatile anesthetic agents. Both propofol anesthesia and inhalational anesthesia are more emetogenic when N_2O is used in combination. There is no difference in emetogenicity between isoflurane, desflurane, and sevoflurane. One of the findings of the International Multicenter Protocol to assess Antiemetic Combinations Trial (IMPACT) was that, by eliminating N_2O as the carrier gas, PONV risk is reduced by about 12%.[6]
3. Minimization of perioperative opioids reduces PONV risk. Infiltration with local anesthetics and the use of alternative nonnarcotic analgesics are opioid sparing. Ketorolac has been available and in use for more than a decade.

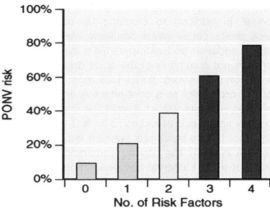

Risk factors	Points
Female gender	1
Nonsmoker	1
History of PONV	1
Postoperative opioids	1
Risk score =	0...4

Fig. 1. Risk factors for developing PONV. (*From* Apfel CC, Läärä E, Koivuranta M, et al. A simplified risk score for predicting postoperative nausea and vomiting: conclusions from cross-validations between two centers. Anesthesiology 1999;91(3):693–700; with permission.)

Some surgeons are reluctant to use it because it causes inhibition of platelet aggregation by inhibiting cyclooxygenase. Although the increased incidence of bleeding is small, when surgical outcome is jeopardized, many surgeons avoid using it.

Intravenous acetaminophen (Ofirmev) was approved by the US Food and Drug Administration (FDA) in late 2010. Most studies of Ofirmev use report less opioid consumption and a lower percentage of patients requiring rescue medications. The rapid blood level achieved by the intravenous route provides an excellent alternative or adjunct for those patients requiring mild to moderate pain relief.

4. Regional anesthesia is associated with a marked reduction in PONV risk compared with general inhalational anesthesia by avoiding exposure to volatile anesthetics and narcotics.

PONV PROPHYLAXIS
Serotonin Antagonists

The serotonin antagonists have become one of the foundation drug classes in the treatment of PONV. Much of what is known about antiemetic prophylaxis has come from therapies effective in chemotherapy-induced nausea and vomiting. Cytotoxic chemotherapy is associated with release of serotonin from the gut. This released serotonin may stimulate vagal afferents in the gut through 5-hydroxytryptamine (5-HT3) receptors and initiate vomiting. Serotonin is also found throughout the central nervous system, including the CTZ.

The 5-HT3 receptor antagonists (5-HT3-RAs) include ondansetron (Zofran), dolasetron (Anzemet), granisetron (Kytril), and, most recently, palonosetron (Aloxi). All are approved for use in the United States. In general, all are considered safe and equally effective. Ondansetron was the first of its class and the most widely studied. The most common side effects (headache, constipation, and diarrhea) occur at a low rate. These drugs are not sedating and do not cause extrapyramidal side effects, which makes them particularly useful.

It is recommended that ondansetron 4 mg (and other drugs in this class) be given 20 to 30 minutes before the end of surgery to provide prophylaxis for 4 to 6 hours after surgery in the case of ondansetron. The variable chemical structures of each of these drugs may explain the minor differences in dose response and duration of action. Palonosetron is unique in this group, with a long half-life of about 40 hours, which may make it useful in the prevention of PDNV.

Steroids

Dexamethasone is effective in the management of PONV. It has a slow onset of action and consequently the recommendation is to administer it immediately following induction of anesthesia. Although the mechanism of action is not completely known, it is thought that steroids inhibit prostaglandin synthesis centrally or lead to endorphin release. The Society for Ambulatory Anesthesia (SAMBA) guidelines endorse the use of 4 to 5 mg of dexamethasone, whereas other studies have determined that higher doses (8 mg) are more effective.[7,8] There seems to be no clinical toxicity associated with the use of dexamethasone for PONV prophylaxis.

Dopamine Antagonists

There are several groups of drugs that are dopamine antagonists. The two most common in the class of butyrophenones are droperidol and halo-peridol. In addition to blocking D_2 receptors, these drugs cause alpha blockade, which can lead to sedation and extrapyramidal symptoms, although not commonly at the small doses given for PONV prophylaxis (0.625/1.25 mg). The efficacy of droperidol as a cost-effective antiemetic has been well established. It would be considered by many anesthesia providers to be first-line therapy if not for the black-box warning imposed by the FDA in 2001. The concern regarding prolongation of the QT interval has been implicated in the development of torsades de pointes; although evidence of this effect with small antiemetic doses is lacking. Most other currently available antiemetics also cause QT prolongation, including the phenothiazines, antihistamines, and the 5-HT3-RA, ondansetron. Hypothermia and the duration of general anesthesia are also associated with QT prolongation. There has been a drastic decline in the use of droperidol since this warning. In our institution, droperidol use is limited to high-risk patients who will have cardiac monitoring for at least 2 hours from the time of drug administration. Although effective, haloperidol can only be given by the intramuscular route because of similar concerns of cardiac dysrhythmia.

The phenothiazines, promethazine (Phenergan) and prochlorperazine (Compazine) are commonly used antiemetics. Because of numerous adverse effects such as agitation, somnolence, and extrapyramidal effects, their use is not considered first-line therapy. A retrospective review comparing the efficacy of a repeat dose of ondansetron for established PONV versus 6.25 mg of promethazine showed greater efficacy with promethazine. Higher doses of promethazine did not increase efficacy.[9] This finding supports the recommendations by experts to choose a drug from another class when the first drug fails, because the receptors targeted by the first drug given are already blocked. The use of intravenous promethazine is associated with a small but serious risk of venous thrombosis and inflammation. It is essential to ensure that promethazine is administered slowly in a well-functioning intravenous line. Although commonly used, Compazine has not been well studied for effectiveness.

The benzamide, metoclopramide, blocks both central and peripheral D_2 receptors. At the commonly used 10-mg dose, numerous studies have failed to show antiemetic efficacy and it is therefore not recommended for PONV prophylaxis.[10] Higher doses may be effective but lead to an unacceptably high incidence of extrapyramidal symptoms.

Antihistamines

Diphenhydramine (Benadryl) is an H_1 blocker with antiemetic effects at the recommended dose of 1 mg/kg intravenously. Its use in PONV prophylaxis has not been well studied. The anticholinergic side effects of dry mouth, blurred vision, and urinary retention limit its use.

Cholinergic Antagonists

Scopolamine and atropine block cholinergic muscarinic emetic receptors in the central nervous system. Because of its weaker antiemetic properties and resultant tachycardia, atropine is not used for PONV prophylaxis. Transdermal scopolamine has been shown to be effective as an antiemetic.[11] Its anticholinergic side effects of blurred vision, dry mouth, and restlessness, as well as its 2-hour to 4-hour onset of action, limit its use. It may be useful in combination with other agents in high-risk patients and in the prevention of PDNV.

MANAGEMENT STRATEGIES

The IMPACT study established that the three most commonly used antiemetics, ondansetron 4 mg, dexamethasone 4 mg, and droperidol 1.25 mg, are equally effective for PONV prophylaxis.[6] Various combinations of these three interventions were examined and each antiemetic was found to act independently and to reduce risk by about 26%. It was also shown that the efficacy of these drugs is primarily dependent on the baseline risk rather than on which antiemetic was given. The first antiemetic has the greatest impact on reducing risk; additional antiemetics in a combination regimen add less and less benefit as the baseline risk decreases, as shown in **Table 1**. Also shown in the table is that those with the greatest risk benefit the most from PONV prophylaxis, whereas those with already low risk, benefit little. For example, a patient with no risk factors has a 10% baseline risk for PONV. If this patient receives 1 intervention, the risk for PONV is reduced only to about 7%, which demonstrates why prophylaxis is not generally recommended in this group of patients (**Fig. 2**).

Low Risk

These patients have 0 to 1 risk factor for PONV. A reasonable approach to these patients is to either use a single antiemetic agent or none at all if the procedure is short, not invasive, and there are no serious medical or surgical consequences to consider. Dexamethasone and the 5-HT3-RA are considered first-line therapy. Because dexamethasone is not immediately effective, it should be

Table 1
Estimated PONV incidence as a function of baseline risk, assuming each intervention reduces relative risk by 26% (values given as %)

	Number of Interventions			
None[a]	One	Two	Three	Four
10	7	5	4	3
20	15	11	8	6
40	29	22	16	12
60	44	33	24	18
80	59	44	32	24

[a] The baseline risk levels of 10%, 20%, 40%, 60%, and 80% reflect 0, 1, 2, 3, and 4 risk factors considered in a simplified risk score.

From Apfel CC, Korttila K, Abdalla M, et al. A factorial trial of six interventions for the prevention of postoperative nausea and vomiting. N Engl J Med 2004;350:2449; with permission.

given following induction. Ondansetron (or other 5-HT3-RAs) are reserved for rescue treatment; this group of drugs is effective for established PONV.[12]

Intermediate Risk

These patients have 2 to 3 risk factors. For example, a nonsmoking woman has 2 risk factors from the outset. Female gender is the strongest risk factor for PONV and the risk persists long after menopause. It is generally recommended that

patients with intermediate risk have at least 2 interventions. These interventions could be either combination antiemetics, such as dexamethasone and a 5-HT3-RA, or a propofol-based anesthetic with dexamethasone. Measures to minimize opioid use, such as the use of local anesthetics when appropriate and nonnarcotic analgesics (Ketorolac or Ofirmev), reduce risk.

If ondansetron (or other 5-HT3-RA) has been used during the course of anesthesia and the patient develops PONV in the PACU (postanesthesia care unit), a drug from another class should be chosen because the serotonin receptors are already blocked. Promethazine at a dose of 6.25 mg may be used as rescue therapy in this case.[9] Droperidol could also be given if the patient can be monitored on a cardiac monitor for 2 hours. A second dose of ondansetron can be given if 4 to 6 hours have passed since the initial dose.

High Risk

Patients with 3 or 4 risk factors require a multimodal approach because no combination of 2 or even 3 antiemetics eliminates the possibility of developing PONV. Scuderi and colleagues[13] introduced the concept of multimodal therapy in high-risk patients, which included propofol and remifentanil intravenous anesthesia (TIVA), dual antiemetic prophylaxis with droperidol (0.625 mg) and dexamethasone (10 mg), ketorolac, hydration with 25 mL/kg total fluids, and 1 mg ondansetron at the end of the case. Only 1 patient required treatment of nausea in

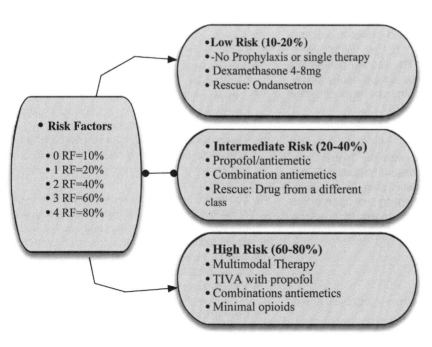

Fig. 2. Risk factors and PONV management strategy.

• **Risk Factors**

• 0 RF=10%
• 1 RF=20%
• 2 RF=40%
• 3 RF=60%
• 4 RF=80%

•**Low Risk (10-20%)**
•-No Prophylaxis or single therapy
• Dexamethasone 4-8mg
• Rescue: Ondansetron

• **Intermediate Risk (20-40%)**
• Propofol/antiemetic
• Combination antiemetics
• Rescue: Drug from a different class

• **High Risk (60-80%)**
• Multimodal Therapy
• TIVA with propofol
• Combinations antiemetics
• Minimal opioids

the PACU and this was treated with 12.5 mg of diphenhydramine. This study was able to show that it is possible to decrease PONV to a low level in high-risk patients but it requires the increased expertise needed to perform TIVA rather than the relative ease of providing general anesthesia with a vaporizer.

PDNV

In a recently published prospective multicenter study of ambulatory surgery patients having general anesthesia, Apfel and colleagues found a remarkably high incidence of 37% for nausea and/or vomiting following discharge. This is in contrast to the approximately 21% of the same group having nausea and/or vomiting in the PACU.[4] They found 5 independent risk factors for PDNV: female gender, age less than 50 years, history of PONV, opioids administered in the PACU, and nausea in the PACU. These risks factors are similar to those found to predict PONV. The most significant finding is that patients who experience nausea in the PACU have a 3-fold higher risk for developing PDNV. Ondansetron administered during surgery and a TIVA with propofol are not protective for PDNV because of the short half-lives of both of these drugs.

The agents or combinations of agents that will prove useful in PDNV prevention remain unclear at this time. In the study by Apfel and colleagues,[4] dexamethasone significantly reduced PDNV. The first FDA-approved neurokinin-1 receptor antagonist aprepitant (Emend) has been found to be superior to ondansetron in the prevention of vomiting in the first 24 to 48 hours following surgery.[14] Aprepitant is well tolerated and comes in oral and intravenous forms that may be useful when other agents have failed. The second-generation 5-HT3-RA palonosetron has a significantly longer half-life than ondansetron and consequently may be efficacious in reducing PDNV.

SUMMARY

Identifying those patients with the highest risk leads to the greatest success in reducing PONV by modifying the anesthetic plan to decrease baseline risk, and implementing the appropriate use of prophylaxis. The strategies that will be effective in the reduction of PDNV are currently under investigation.

REFERENCES

1. Kapur PA. The big "little problem" [editorial]. Anesth Analg 1991;73:243–5.
2. Gan T, Sloan F, Dear G, et al. How much are patients willing to pay to avoid postoperative nausea and vomiting? Anesth Analg 2001;92:393–400.
3. Gan TJ, Meyer T, Apfel CC, et al. Consensus guidelines for managing postoperative nausea and vomiting. Anesth Analg 2003;97:62–71.
4. Apfel CC, Philip BK, Cakmakkaya OS, et al. Who is at risk for postoperative nausea and vomiting after ambulatory surgery? Anesthesiology 2012;117: 475–86.
5. Apfel CC, Läärä E, Koivuranta M, et al. A simplified risk score for predicting postoperative nausea and vomiting: conclusions from cross-validations between two centers. Anesthesiology 1999;91(3): 693–700.
6. Apfel CC, Korttila K, Abdalla M, et al. A factorial trial of six interventions for the prevention of postoperative nausea and vomiting. N Engl J Med 2004;350: 2441–51.
7. Gan TJ, Meyer T, Apfel CC, et al. Society for ambulatory anesthesia guidelines for the management of postoperative nausea and vomiting. Anesth Analg 2007;105:1615–28.
8. Elhakim M, Nafie M, Mahmoud K, et al. Dexamethasone 8 mg in combination with ondansetron 4 mg appears to be the optimal dose for the prevention of nausea and vomiting after laparoscopic cholecystectomy. Can J Anaesth 2002; 49(9):922–6.
9. Habib AS, Reuveni J, Taguchi A, et al. A comparison of ondansetron with promethazine for treating postoperative nausea and vomiting in patients who received prophylaxis with ondansetron: a retrospective database analysis. Anesth Analg 2007;104(3): 548–51.
10. Henzi I, Walder B, Tramer MR. Metochlopramide in the preventions of postoperative nausea and vomiting: a quantitative systematic review of randomized placebo-controlled studies. Br J Anaesth 1999; 83(5):761–71.
11. Carlisle J, Stevenson C. Drugs for preventing postoperative nausea and vomiting. Cochrane Database Syst Rev 2006;(3):CD004125.
12. Kazemi-Kjellberg F, Henzi I, Tramer MR. Treatment of established postoperative nausea and vomiting: a quantitative systematic review. BMC Anesthesiol 2001;1(1):2.
13. Scuderi PE, James RL, Harris L, et al. Multimodal Antiemetic Management Prevents Early Postoperative Vomiting After Outpatient Laparoscopy. Anesth Analg 2000;91(6):1408–14.
14. Gan TJ, Apfel CC, Kovac A, et al. A randomized, double-blind comparison of the NK1 antagonist, aprepitant, versus ondansetron for the prevention of postoperative nausea and vomiting. Anesth Analg 2007;105(5):1082–9.

Evidence-based Medicine and Data Sharing in Outpatient Plastic Surgery

Geoffrey R. Keyes, MD[a,b,*], Foad Nahai, MD[c], Ronald E. Iverson, MD[d,e], Robert Singer, MD[f,g]

KEYWORDS

- Evidence-based medicine • Data sharing • Outpatient surgery • Plastic surgery
- Patient outcomes • EBM implementation

KEY POINTS

- Plastic surgery organizations have put forth initiatives to improve EBM skills among plastic surgeons.
- Small steps toward understanding and mastering the practice increase the level of expertise, improve outcomes for patients, and raise the bar for patient safety.
- Openness toward data sharing and better standards for implementing it strengthen the evidence base and lead to better health care quality and optimal patient outcomes.
- Modern EBM is composed of five core steps: (1) assessing clinical practice to identify an important patient or policy problem; (2) asking clinical questions that are related to the problem and constructed to facilitate a sufficient literature search; (3) acquiring the best available evidence to answer the clinical question; (4) appraising the validity, importance, and clinical use of the evidence; and (5) applying evidence that is relevant to individual patients and aligned with their preferences and values.

INTRODUCTION

To become a plastic and reconstructive surgeon requires years of graduated responsibility in a structured residency training program. During this training period prospective surgeons gain technical expertise to perform surgical procedures and manage patient care through careful observation of their mentors and increasing responsibility, much like an apprenticeship.[1] Although the mentors are incredibly skilled and experts in their field, relying on expert opinion to make treatment decisions is no longer sufficient in the realm of evidence-based medicine (EBM). As pressures from regulators and payers are increasing, the performance of surgeons is being scrutinized like never before. Treatment decisions that were once based on various forms of evidence, such as years of surgical practice, successes with previous patients, and information from the surgical literature, must now be supported by strong clinical evidence to be considered acceptable by the wider health care community.[1]

Plastic surgeons must be dedicated to patient safety and quality improvement in all areas of practice. The use of EBM is particularly important for outpatient surgery, because approximately

[a] Accreditation of Ambulatory Surgery Facilities, Inc (AAAASF), PO Box 9500, 5101 Washington Street, 2F Gurnee, IL 60031, USA; [b] Department of Plastic Surgery, Keck School of Medicine, University of Southern California, Los Angeles, California, USA; [c] Emory University School of Medicine, Atlanta, Georgia; [d] Stanford University Medical School, Palo Alto, California; [e] American Association for the Accreditation of Surgical Facilities, Illinois, USA; [f] University of California, San Diego, USA; [g] American Association for Accreditation of Ambulatory Surgery Facilities, Inc (AAAASF), La Jolla, California, USA
* Corresponding author.
E-mail address: geoffreykeyes@sbcglobal.net

Clin Plastic Surg 40 (2013) 453–463
http://dx.doi.org/10.1016/j.cps.2013.04.008

80% of surgeries in the United States are performed as outpatient procedures[2] and many ambulatory surgery facilities are unaccredited and in many states uninspected, with no regulatory oversight.[3] Efforts are underway to promote accreditation of ambulatory surgery centers,[3] but learning EBM and implementing its principles are also critical for improving quality and patient outcomes in the outpatient setting.

HISTORY AND PRINCIPLES OF EBM

EBM is the conscientious, explicit, and judicious use of current best evidence, combined with individual clinical expertise and patient preferences and values, in making decisions about the care of individual patients.[4] Rudimentary accounts of evidence-based practice date back to ancient times[5,6]; however, the term "evidence-based medicine" did not exist until the early 1990s, when it was first published in the ACP Journal Club[7] and later introduced to the wider medical community by the Evidence-Based Medicine Working Group.[8] Initially, the concept of EBM was met with much criticism, because it incorrectly implied that the practice of medicine was unscientific. Over time, health care professionals began to understand that EBM was a framework and cultural standard for finding and applying the best evidence to guide treatment decisions.[9]

Although the acceptance and practice of EBM has increased since the early 1990s, audits of medical and surgical procedures have revealed that low levels of evidence are still guiding treatment decisions.[10–12] Importantly, these audits were conducted at single institutions shortly after EBM emerged, so it is unclear if the findings are representative of most health care facilities today. Nevertheless, there are always be cases for which little to no evidence is available, and clinicians need to rely on their best judgment and best available evidence at the time, but more work is needed to increase awareness of EBM and promote better research practices to enhance the evidence base and ensure that most treatment decisions are based on sound evidence.

Unfortunately, even when evidence is available, the research findings have the potential to be biased. This bias, or systematic error, is a reproducible error in study design or conduct that leads to systematic deviations from the underlying truth.[9,13] Basing treatment decisions on biased information or inadequately tested theories can have devastating effects on patient outcomes.[14] Therefore, clinicians need an understanding of EBM principles to help identify the best evidence to guide practice.

Modern EBM is composed of five core steps: (1) assessing clinical practice to identify an important patient or policy problem; (2) asking clinical questions that are related to the problem and constructed to facilitate a sufficient literature search; (3) acquiring the best available evidence to answer the clinical question; (4) appraising the validity, importance, and clinical use of the evidence; and (5) applying evidence that is relevant to individual patients and aligned with their preferences and values.[9,15] **Table 1** provides an overview of these steps and helpful methods for accomplishing each step, which are also described herein.

After a problem has been identified, developing a good clinical question facilitates a successful literature search. Clinical questions can be about treatment; harm; prognosis; diagnosis; or cost-effectiveness (economic analysis). The PICO (Population, Intervention, Comparison, Outcome) method is commonly used to develop clinical questions.[9,15] An answerable clinical question in outpatient plastic surgery may be: "For women with breast hypertrophy, does breast reduction compared with physical therapy result in better health-related quality of life?," where the patient population is women with breast hypertrophy, the intervention is breast reduction, the comparison intervention is physical therapy, and the outcome is health-related quality of life.

Finding the evidence to answer the clinical question involves several steps. First is to define the literature search strategy. The STARLITE (Sampling strategy, Type of study, Approaches, Limits, Inclusion/exclusion criteria, Terms, and Electronic sources) method is a useful tool for developing a search strategy.[16] The type of clinical question helps to narrow the search to specific types of studies. For example, clinical questions about therapy are best answered with data from randomized controlled trials (RCTs), whereas clinical questions about prognosis are best answered with data from cohort designs. All types of study designs can be included in the search to optimize results, especially when little evidence exists for a particular question or a particular study design is not feasible or ethical; however, searches should aim to identify studies with the highest levels of evidence to best inform clinical decisions. Searching several bibliographic databases, including repositories of gray literature, and hand searching the bibliographies of relevant articles increases the likelihood that the body of evidence that has been collected is comprehensive and represents the underlying truth.

A common misconception in EBM is that the study design alone determines the strength of the evidence. Although RCTs can provide strong evidence, they are not created equal. The results

Table 1
Core steps of EBM and methods for performing each step

Step	Description	Methods
Assess	Recognize, classify, and prioritize important patient or policy problems	Assess problems in individual practice Search review articles and clinical practice guidelines to identify unmet medical needs Discuss areas of interest and potential clinical issues with colleagues Listen to patients to identify unmet needs that are important to patients
Ask	Construct clinical questions that facilitate an efficient search for evidence	Use PICO to develop good clinical questions: identify the patient/population/problem, intervention, comparison, outcomes
Acquire	Gather important and convincing evidence from high-quality repositories of the health literature	Use STARTLITE to develop a search strategy. Identify the: Sampling strategy: all or selected studies Type of study: systematic reviews, RCT, and so forth Approaches: electronic search, hand search, and so forth Limits: English-language articles, humans, age of patients Inclusion and exclusion: criteria for including or excluding studies Terms: search terms (MeSH terms, key words, and so forth) Electronic sources: electronic databases (eg, MEDLINE, CINAHL, Cochrane Library, and so forth)
Appraise	Systematically check best available evidence for indications of validity, importance, and usefulness	Use critical appraisal tools and resources to assess for potential biases: Center for Evidence Based Medicine, http://www.cebm.net/ Users' Guides to the Medical Literature (JAMAevidence), http://jamaevidence.com/ Critical Appraisal Skills Program, http://www.casp-uk.net/ Grading of Recommendations Assessment Development and Evaluation Working Group http://www.gradeworkinggroup.org/index.htm
Apply	Interpret the applicability of evidence to specific problems, given patient preferences and values	Weigh the risks and benefits of the treatment option for each patient Ensure that the treatment option aligns with the patient's values and preferences Develop plans for implementing the evidence in private practice and larger health care facilities (knowledge translation)

of small, poorly designed RCTs can be misleading. Therefore, all types of studies should be appraised to determine their validity, importance, and clinical applicability. Critical appraisal is the process by which the methodologic quality of a study is screened for potential biases. Several critical appraisal tools have been developed to aid clinicians with this process. Importantly, each type of study is evaluated by a specific set of criteria. **Box 1** provides an example of a critical appraisal tool for evaluating an RCT.

If after critical appraisal the study is deemed to be of high quality for the particular study design, it is then assigned a level of evidence according to the clinical question that the study attempted to answer. Numerous rating scales and their iterations have been published over the years; many are based on the first rating scale that was published by the Canadian Task Force[17] and later refined by Sackett[18] and the Center for Evidence Based Medicine.[19] Typically, levels of evidence range from I to V, with I representing the highest

> **Box 1**
> **Critical appraisal tool for an RCT**
>
> *Assessment for Selection Bias*
> - Where patients recruited appropriately?
> - Was allocation concealed?
> - Were participants randomized appropriately?
> - Were treatment groups similar with respect to known and unknown prognostic factors?
> - Were confounders addressed?
> - Were data complete for at least 80% of participants in each group?
> - Were any significant differences found between participants who were lost to follow-up and those who completed follow-up?
> - Were participants analyzed in the group to which they were randomized (intention-to-treat)?
>
> *Assessment for Intervention Bias*
> - Was the intervention well described?
> - Was the intervention implemented similarly in all participants (ie, could level of surgeon expertise influence how the procedure was performed; were there any protocol deviations)?
> - Was the caregiver (eg, surgeon) masked?
>
> *Assessment for Measurement Bias*
> - Were the participants, outcome assessors, and data analysts masked?
> - Were outcomes measured similarly and with valid, defined criteria?
> - Was follow-up sufficient to detect all outcomes of interest?
>
> *Assessment for Type II Error*
> - Was power sufficient to detect differences for each measured outcome?

level or strongest evidence and V representing the lowest level or weakest evidence. *Plastic and Reconstructive Surgery* has implemented a pyramid system to identify the clinical question and level of evidence of studies published in the journal (**Fig. 1**).[20] The pyramid is located on the first page of each article, providing a prominent visual cue that alerts the reader to the strength of the evidence provided by the study.

After critically appraising each study for a particular clinical question, the collective body of evidence is graded according to its strength in guiding a clinical recommendation. Like rating scales for levels of evidence, a variety of grading scales are available for recommendations. Recommendations are typically graded from A to D, with A representing the strongest recommendation and D representing the weakest recommendation. High levels of evidence often lead to strong clinical recommendations; however, this is not always the case. For example, high-level evidence suggests that continuous anticoagulation therapy reduces the risk of recurrent thrombosis in patients who have had an unprovoked deep vein thrombosis. However, continuous treatment with an anticoagulant also increases the risk of bleeding and is inconvenient for the patient. Therefore, weighing the benefits and risks of continuous anticoagulation therapy for this patient population may result in only a weak to moderate recommendation.[21] **Tables 2** and **3** illustrate the evidence and recommendation scales used by the American Society of Plastic Surgeons and the American Society of Aesthetic Plastic Surgery.[22,23]

Although scales for rating the level of evidence and grading recommendations are largely similar across medical specialties, a universally accepted rating system has yet to be established. The Grading of Recommendations Assessment Development and Evaluation Working Group, an international collaboration of experts in EBM, is focused on addressing concerns with the current grading systems in health care and has developed its own approach to evaluating evidence and recommendations that is gaining acceptance worldwide.[24]

CURRENT IMPLEMENTATION OF EBM

Today, EBM is used in many ways to guide practice. Individual clinicians, guideline developers, and CME providers use EBM to identify and teach best practices. The US Food and Drug Administration and other regulatory agencies worldwide require strong clinical evidence to approve new drugs and devices.[25] With increasing demands to fulfill unmet medical needs, regulatory agencies will likely tighten regulatory requirements regarding evidence. Government and private health plans also use evidence to determine the value and cost effectiveness of therapeutic products and develop reimbursement schedules for such treatments. EBM is the foundation for comparative effectiveness research (CER), which was introduced by the Congressional Budget Office in 2007[26] and later redefined by the Federal Coordinating Council for CER "...to improve health outcomes by developing and disseminating evidence-based information to patients, clinicians, and other decision-makers, responding to their expressed needs, about which interventions are most

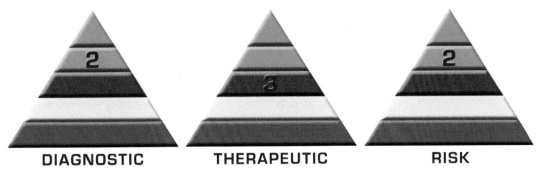

Fig. 1. Levels of evidence pyramid identifying the clinical question and level of evidence (I through V) of studies published in *Plastic and Reconstructive Surgery*. (*Left*) Diagnostic clinical question addressed, with a level of evidence of II. (*Center*) Therapeutic clinical question addressed, with a level of evidence of III. (*Right*) Risk clinical question addressed, with a level of evidence of II. (*From* Sullivan D, Chung KC, Eaves FF, et al. The level of evidence pyramid: indicating levels of evidence in *Plastic and Reconstructive Surgery* articles. Plast Reconstr Surg 2011;128:311–4; with permission.)

effective for which patients under specific circumstances."[27] CER promotes the use of EBM to address practical clinical questions in real-world settings to identify optimal treatments for individual patients. Although RCTs and meta-analyses are still predominant components in CER, other sources of evidence, such as observational studies, registry data, and health-related quality-of-life studies, are considered because they complement randomized studies and contribute to the larger body of evidence that may help to identify important patient needs.

Patient values and preferences are important components of EBM.[9] In 2010, Congress developed the Patient Centered Outcomes Research Institute (PCORI) through the Patient Protection and Affordable Care Act to facilitate comparative clinical effectiveness research. Although developed by Congress, PCORI is an independent organization with a Board of Governors comprised of 21 members who represent all stakeholders. EBM is central to PCORI's goals and is emphasized in its mission statement: "[PCORI] helps people make informed health care decisions—and improves health care delivery and outcomes—by producing and promoting high integrity, evidence-based information that comes from research guided by patients, caregivers and the broader health care community."[28] It is unclear how this initiative will change in the coming years, but EBM will almost certainly remain a strong component in health care legislation and regulation moving forward.

EVIDENCE-BASED PLASTIC SURGERY: CHALLENGES AND SOLUTIONS

Plastic surgery organizations, such as the American Society of Plastic Surgeons and American Society of Aesthetic Plastic Surgery, have set forth initiatives to promote awareness of EBM in plastic surgery and to teach its principles to the practicing surgeon[23,29–33]; however, surgeons may be hesitant to adopt EBM practices because of time constraints, limited surgical evidence, and inherent challenges in designing rigorous surgical studies.

Table 2 Scale for rating the level of evidence of therapeutic studies[a]	
Level of Evidence	Qualifying Studies
I	High-quality, multicentered or single-centered, randomized controlled trial with adequate power; or systematic review of these studies
II	Lesser-quality, randomized controlled trial; prospective cohort or comparative study; or systematic review of these studies
III	Retrospective cohort or comparative study, case-control study, or systematic review of these studies
IV	Case series with pretest and posttest, or only posttest
V	Expert opinion developed by consensus process; case report or clinical example; or evidence based on physiology, bench research, or "first principles"

[a] Scales for rating prognostic and diagnostic studies differ from this scale.

Table 3
Scale for grading recommendations

Grade	Descriptor	Qualifying Evidence	Implications for Practice
A	Strong recommendation	Level I evidence or consistent findings from multiple studies of levels II, III, or IV	Clinicians should follow a strong recommendation unless a clear and compelling rationale for an alternative approach is present
B	Recommendation	Levels II, III, or IV evidence and findings are generally consistent	Generally, clinicians should follow a recommendation but should remain alert to new information and sensitive to patient preferences
C	Option	Levels II, III, or IV evidence, but findings are inconsistent	Clinicians should be flexible in their decision-making regarding appropriate practice, although they may set bounds on alternatives; patient preference should have a substantial influencing role
D	Option	Level V: little or no systematic empiric evidence	Clinicians should consider all options in their decision-making and be alert to new published evidence that clarifies the balance of benefit vs harm; patient preference should have a substantial influencing role

Unlike medicine, surgical procedures are often difficult to evaluate with RCTs; according to data from a systematic review on surgical studies, only 40% of the clinical questions could be answered with a randomized study design.[34] As a result, most surgical studies are retrospective case series or reports.[1,13,35,36] Although designing surgical trials may be challenging, attention to good research design may help to improve the surgical evidence base. Surgical trials that are not randomized are subject to selection bias, which occurs when treatment groups are different with respect to known and unknown prognostic factors. If baseline characteristics are not well balanced between the groups, it becomes less clear that any differences in outcomes between the treatment groups are associated with the intervention. Because randomization in surgical studies is not always feasible or ethical, researchers must minimize potential bias in other ways. Inclusion and exclusion criteria can be used to ensure that the study population is comprised of patients with similar characteristics. Another option is matching each patient in one group to a patient in the other group who has similar prognostic factors. Additionally, statistical methods that account for potential confounders (eg, multivariate analyses) should be defined a priori and incorporated into data analysis to determine the effects of known confounders on patient outcomes. Although these strategies can minimize selection bias in the absence of randomization, they are unable to eliminate the potential effects of unknown confounders.[13]

When blinding (or masking) is not incorporated into the study design and individuals involved in the study are aware of the treatment allocation, intervention and measurement biases can occur. In surgical trials, masking of surgeons is usually impossible, but masking of other individuals, such as patients, other health care providers, outcome assessors, and data analysts, should be attempted whenever feasible to minimize potential biases.[13] Surgeon expertise and preferences also can introduce intervention bias into surgical studies. Allowing time for surgeons to master the surgical intervention before initiating the study and using expertise-based RCTs, where patients are randomized to a surgeon instead of a treatment arm, can help to overcome potential biases associated with differential expertise among the investigators.[1,13]

Measurement bias can occur when outcome assessors are not masked to treatment allocation or when outcomes are not well defined or measured with standardized criteria. Therefore, defining clinical end points and outcome measures a priori is extremely important. Objective outcomes, especially those that are indisputable (eg, mortality), are less likely to introduce measurement bias; however, outcomes in plastic surgery are often subjective (eg, cosmesis, quality of life, or patient satisfaction).[13] Investigators should incorporate objective measures whenever possible. For example, in studies that aim to determine the rate of infection after a surgical procedure, "infection" should be well defined and diagnosed with a standardized set of criteria (eg, Centers for Disease Control and Prevention Surgical Site Infection [SSI])[37] during the study. Efforts are underway to develop validated tools for measuring other outcomes, such as health-related quality of life after plastic surgery.[38]

Determining the minimum amount of follow-up is important for ensuring that all outcomes of interest are detected during the study.[13] Similar to the previous scenario, if SSI is an outcome of interest, then follow-up should be at least 30 days according to the Centers for Disease Control and Prevention's definition of SSIs.[37] Losses to follow-up should also be accounted for in data analysis, because patients who fail to complete follow-up may be different from those who do, and those differences may influence the study results.[13]

Attention must also be paid to other elements of study design, such as determining the required sample size (ie, performing power calculations a priori) and incorporating intention-to-treat analyses to increase validity of study results.[13] Research reporting guidelines are helpful for designing clinical trials and ensuring that methods

and results are reported properly. Guidelines for various types of study designs (eg, CONSORT for RCTs) are available on the Web site of the EQUATOR Network.[39]

THE ROLE OF DATA SHARING IN EBM AND ITS IMPORTANCE FOR IMPROVING HEALTH CARE QUALITY AND PATIENT OUTCOMES

Data sharing is particularly critical to the implementation of EBM. Restricted access to research data precludes a thorough evaluation of all evidence for a particular clinical question, potentially leading to reporting bias and erroneous conclusions about therapeutic interventions and other health care issues. Publication bias is a form of reporting bias that occurs when the publication of a study depends on the direction and statistical significance of the study results. For example, studies with positive findings are published more frequently than those with negative findings. An audit of more than 30,000 surgery articles from 12 journals revealed that 74% of the articles reported positive findings, 9% were neutral, and only 17% reported negative findings.[40] Publication bias and other forms of reporting bias (**Table 4**)[41] can threaten the validity of studies that synthesize large amounts of data, such as meta-analyses.[42–44] If access to data is restricted and investigators fail to sufficiently search the gray literature for unpublished data, the results of meta-analyses may be inaccurate. According to a survey of recent meta-analyses of RCTs,

Table 4
Types of reporting bias

Type of Reporting Bias	Definition
Publication bias	The *publication* or *non-publication* of research findings, depending on the nature and direction of the results
Time lag bias	The *rapid* or *delayed* publication of research findings, depending on the nature and direction of the results
Multiple (duplicate) publication bias	The *multiple* or *singular* publication of research findings, depending on the nature and direction of the results
Location bias	The publication of research findings in journals with different *ease of access* or *levels of indexing* in standard databases, depending on the nature and direction of results
Citation bias	The *citation* or *non-citation* of research findings, depending on the nature and direction of the results
Language bias	The publication of research findings *in a particular language*, depending on the nature and direction of the results
Outcome reporting bias	The *selective reporting* of some outcomes but not others, depending on the nature and direction of the results

From Higgins JP, Green S, editors. Cochrane handbook for systematic reviews of interventions version 5.1.0 [updated March 2011]. The Cochrane Collaboration. 2011. Available at: www.cochrane-handbook.org. Accessed October 12, 2012; with permission.

only 29% of the meta-analyses included data from gray literature.[42] In another study in which investigators re-evaluated meta-analyses of drug trials by incorporating unpublished data that were not included in the original meta-analyses, 46% of the re-evaluated meta-analyses showed lower efficacy, 46% showed greater efficacy, and only 7% showed identical efficacy compared with the original meta-analyses.[45] Complete reporting, data sharing, and transparency in research are needed to ensure that the published body of evidence represents the truth.

Several government agencies, organizations, foundations, journal editors, and other entities worldwide are promoting the importance of data sharing for improving health care quality and patient outcomes. In the United States, the Health Information Technology for Economic and Clinical Health Act promotes the use of digital technology to provide health care professionals with critical information to improve the quality of care delivery, reduce errors, and decrease costs and to improve population health by simplifying collection, aggregation, and analysis of anonymized health information.[46] The National Institutes of Health mandated that the results of all studies funded by the National Institutes of Health be made publicly available within 12 months of publishing the final, peer-reviewed manuscript.[47] The Bill and Melinda Gates Foundation published its Global Health Data Access Principles,[48] promoting rapid, global access to health-related data to improve the discovery and development of life-saving interventions.

Although there are many compelling reasons for data sharing, there are also significant concerns. Public access to individual patient data poses a risk to patient confidentiality. Albeit small, the risk of inadvertent publication of personal information exists. Even if data are anonymized, patients could be identified, especially those with rare conditions or diseases. Moreover, universally accepted definitions of "anonymized" or "deidentified" data remain to be established[49]; thus, information that is protected by one entity may not be protected by others. For example, the Health Insurance Portability and Accountability Act in the United States and the Data Protection Act in the United Kingdom have different definitions of personal information and different provisions for protection.[50,51] Another concern surrounding data sharing is that the unrestricted access to full datasets could lead to publication and promotion of misleading information, potentially causing public health scares with devastating consequences (eg, patients discontinuing treatment or refusing vaccination).[52]

Strategies to minimize the risks associated with data sharing are necessary for improving access to data. Guidelines for publishing raw data and developing and using patient registries are available,[49,53] but universally agreed-upon standards are needed to gain greater acceptance by patients and the wider health care community. Studies have found that patients are often willing to share their health data, but remain concerned about the protection and use of their information and their options for sharing the information.[54,55] Allowing patients to select options for sharing their data and developing effective, universally accepted provisions for protecting and using patient data may increase access to data. Increased resources for implementation are also necessary, because activities involved in data sharing may be time intensive and require effective oversight.[46,52] Additionally, sharing negative study results is essential for ensuring that the evidence base is comprehensive and representative of the truth. Academic institutions, journals, and funding agencies should encourage investigators to publish positive and negative study results.[56]

Outcomes for outpatient surgical procedures, collected through the American Association for Accreditation for Ambulatory Surgery Facilities' Internet Based Quality Assurance Program, have been previously reported.[57,58] Although of great value, outcomes alone do not provide complete information about the surgical process. Care delivery can be improved by inclusion of key elements that led to the outcome. A new concept, originating from the work being done by Keyes and colleagues[57,58] in the area of data collection on outpatient surgery, involves the digitalization of the entire surgical process for individual procedures. Beginning with the indications for surgery and following the delivery of care in the preoperative, intraoperative, and postoperative phases, a digital representation of specific aspects of care is integrated with outcomes, which can help identify the root causes for the outcomes, rather than just identifying the outcomes. This digitalization enhances the ability to provide EBM for specific procedures, improving patient care. For example, identifying the key elements potentially responsible for the development of a venous thromboembolism facilitates the decision to provide chemoprophylaxis.

SUMMARY

Acceptance and implementation of EBM has increased in recent years. Plastic surgery organizations have put forth initiatives to improve EBM skills among plastic surgeons. As plastic surgeons have learned throughout medical school, residency, and their own practices, repetition is the key to mastering skills. EBM is no different. The steps involved in EBM may seem daunting to the busy clinician, but small steps toward understanding and mastering the practice increase the level of expertise, improve outcomes for patients, and raise the bar for patient safety. Designing rigorous surgical studies by incorporating strategies for minimizing bias provides stronger evidence in plastic surgery, and publishing positive and negative findings allows for unbiased analyses of the larger body of evidence. Openness toward data sharing and better standards for implementing it strengthens the evidence base and leads to better health care quality and optimal patient outcomes. Implementing EBM and methods for data sharing in plastic surgery also enhances quality and safety in the outpatient setting.

ACKNOWLEDGMENTS

The authors thank Jennifer Swanson of JS Medical Communications, LLC, for her assistance with the preparation of this manuscript.

REFERENCES

1. McCarthy CM, Collins ED, Pusic AL. Where do we find the best evidence? Plast Reconstr Surg 2008; 122:1942–7.
2. Pasternak LR. Preanesthesia evaluation and testing. In: Twersky RS, Philip BK, editors. Handbook of ambulatory anesthesia. 2nd edition. New York: Springer; 2008. p. 1–23.
3. The American Association for Accreditation of Ambulatory Surgery Facilities. 2012. Available at: http://www.aaaasf.org/pub/site/index.html. Accessed October 11, 2012.
4. Sackett DL, Rosenberg WM, Gray JA, et al. Evidence based medicine: what it is and what it isn't. BMJ 1996;312:71–2.
5. Claridge JA, Fabian TC. History and development of evidence-based medicine. World J Surg 2005; 29:547–53.
6. Doherty S. History of evidence-based medicine: oranges, chloride of lime and leeches. Barriers to teaching old dogs new tricks. Emerg Med Australas 2005;17:314–21.
7. Guyatt G. Evidence-based medicine. ACP J Club (Ann Intern Med) 1991;114(Suppl 2):A-16.
8. The Evidence-Based Medicine Working Group. Evidence-based medicine: a new approach to teaching the practice of medicine. JAMA 1992;268:2420–5.
9. The Evidence-Based Medicine Working Group. Users' guides to the medical literature: essentials of evidence-based clinical practice. Chicago: American Medical Association; 2002.
10. Ellis J, Mulligan I, Rowe J, et al. Inpatient general medicine is evidence based: a-team, Nuffield Department of Clinical Medicine. Lancet 1995; 346:407–10.
11. Howes N, Chagla L, Thorpe M, et al. Surgical practice is evidence based. Br J Surg 1997;84:1220–3.
12. Kingston R, Barry M, Tierney S, et al. Treatment of surgical patients is evidence-based. Eur J Surg 2001;167:324–30.
13. Farrokhyar F, Karanicolas PJ, Thoma A, et al. Randomized controlled trials of surgical interventions. Ann Surg 2010;251:409–16.
14. Evans I, Thornton H, Chalmers I. Testing treatments: better research for better healthcare. London: The British Library; 2006.
15. American Medical Association. Core topics in evidence-based medicine. 2012. Available at: http://www.jamaevidence.com/index. Accessed October 11, 2012.
16. Booth A. "Brimful of STARLITE": toward standards for reporting literature searches. J Med Libr Assoc 2006;94:421–9 e205.
17. Canadian Task Force on the periodic health examination. The periodic health examination. Can Med Assoc J 1979;121:1193–254.
18. Sackett DL. Rules of evidence and clinical recommendations on the use of antithrombotic agents. Chest 1989;95(Suppl 2):2S–4S.
19. OCEBM Levels of Evidence Working Group. The Oxford 2011 levels of evidence. Oxford Centre for Evidence-Based Medicine. Available at: http://www.cebm.net/index.aspx?o=5653. Accessed October 24, 2012.
20. Sullivan D, Chung KC, Eaves FF, et al. The level of evidence pyramid: indicating levels of evidence in Plastic and Reconstructive Surgery articles. Plast Reconstr Surg 2011;128:311–4.
21. Balshem H, Helfand M, Schünemann HJ, et al. GRADE guidelines: 3. Rating the quality of evidence. J Clin Epidemiol 2011;64:401–6.
22. American Society of Plastic Surgeons. Evidence-based clinical practice guidelines. Available at: http://www.plasticsurgery.org/For-Medical-Professionals/Legislation-and-Advocacy/Health-Policy-Resources/Evidence-based-GuidelinesPractice-Parameters/Description-and-Development-of-Evidence-based-Practice-Guidelines.html. Accessed October 24, 2012.
23. Eaves FF, Rohrich RJ. So you want to be an evidence-based plastic surgeon? A lifelong journey. Aesthet Surg J 2011;31:137–42.
24. Guyatt GH, Oxman AD, Vist GE, et al. GRADE: an emerging consensus on rating quality of evidence and strength of recommendations. BMJ 2008;336: 924–6.

25. United States Food and Drug Administration. Pathway to global product safety and quality. Available at: http://www.fda.gov/AboutFDA/CentersOffices/OfficeofGlobalRegulatoryOperationsandPolicy/GlobalProductPathway/default.htm. Accessed October 17, 2012.

26. The Congress of the United States, Congressional Budget Office. Research on the comparative effectiveness of medical treatments: issues and options for an expanded federal role. 2007. Available at: http://www.cbo.gov/sites/default/files/cbofiles/ftpdocs/88xx/doc8891/12-18-comparativeeffectiveness.pdf. Accessed October 11, 2012.

27. Federal Coordinating Council for Comparative Effectiveness Research. Report to the president and congress. 2009. Available at: http://www.hhs.gov/recovery/programs/cer/cerannualrpt.pdf. Accessed October 11, 2012.

28. Patient Centered Outcomes Research Institute. Mission and vision. Available at: http://www.pcori.org/about/mission-and-vision/. Accessed October 11, 2012.

29. Chung KC, Swanson JA, Schmitz D, et al. Introducing evidence-based medicine to plastic and reconstructive surgery. Plast Reconstr Surg 2009;123:1385–9.

30. Swanson JA, Schmitz D, Chung KC. How to practice evidence-based medicine. Plast Reconstr Surg 2010;126:286–94.

31. Eaves FF. Got evidence? Stem cells, bias, and the level of evidence ladder: commentary on: ASAPS/ASPS Position Statement on Stem Cells and Fat Grafting. Aesthet Surg J 2011;31:718–22.

32. Nahai F. Evidence-based medicine in aesthetic surgery. Aesthet Surg J 2011;31:135–6.

33. Eaves F, Pusic AL. Why evidence-based medicine matters to aesthetic surgery. Aesthet Surg J 2012;32:117–9.

34. Solomon MJ, McLeod RS. Should we be performing more randomized controlled trials evaluating surgical operations? Surgery 1995;118:459–67.

35. Loiselle F, Mahabir RC, Harrop AR. Levels of evidence in plastic surgery research over 20 years. Plast Reconstr Surg 2008;121:207e–11e.

36. Chang EY, Pannucci CJ, Wilkins EG. Quality of clinical studies in aesthetic surgery journals: a 10-year review. Aesthet Surg J 2009;29:144–7.

37. Centers for Disease Control. Surgical site infection (SSI) event. 2012. Available at: http://www.cdc.gov/nhsn/psc_pa.html. Accessed October 11, 2012.

38. Cano SJ, Klassen AF, Scott AM, et al. The BREAST-Q: further validation in independent clinical samples. Plast Reconstr Surg 2012;129:293–302.

39. EQUATOR Network. Introduction to reporting guidelines. Available at: http://www.equator-network.org/index.aspx?o=1032. Accessed October 12, 2012.

40. Hasenboehler EA, Choudhry IK, Newman JT, et al. Bias towards publishing positive results in orthopedic and general surgery: a patient safety issue? Patient Saf Surg 2007;1:4.

41. Higgins JP, Green S, editors. Cochrane handbook for systematic reviews of interventions version 5.1.0 [updated March 2011]. The Cochrane Collaboration. 2011. Available at: www.cochrane-handbook.org. Accessed October 12, 2012.

42. Ahmed I, Sutton AJ, Riley RD. Assessment of publication bias, selection bias, and unavailable data in meta-analyses using individual participant data: a database survey. BMJ 2012;344:d7762.

43. McGaursan N, Wieseler B, Kreis J, et al. Reporting bias in medical research: a narrative review. Trials 2010;11:37. Available at: http://www.trialsjournal.com/content/11/1/37. Accessed October 24, 2012.

44. Song F, Parekh S, Hooper L, et al. Dissemination and publication of research findings: an updated review of related biases. Health Technol Assess 2010;14. Available at: http://www.hta.ac.uk/project/1627.asp. Accessed October 24, 2012.

45. Hart B, Lundh A, Bero L. Effect of reporting bias on meta-analyses of drug trials: reanalysis of meta-analyses. BMJ 2011;344:d7202.

46. Public Law 111-5. American Recovery and Reinvestment Act of 2009. Available at: http://www.gpo.gov/fdsys/pkg/PLAW-111publ5/content-detail.html. Accessed October 24, 2012.

47. National Institutes of Health. Revised policy on enhancing public access to archived publications resulting from NIH-funded research. 2009. Available at: http://grants.nih.gov/grants/guide/notice-files/NOT-OD-08-033.html. Accessed October 9, 2012.

48. Bill and Melinda Gates Foundation. Global health data access principles. Available at: http://www.gatesfoundation.org/. Accessed October 25, 2012.

49. Hrynaszkiewicz I, Altman DG. Towards agreement on best practice for publishing raw clinical trial data. Trials 2009;10:17. Available at: http://www.trialsjournal.com/content/10/1/17. Accessed October 9, 2012.

50. United States Department of Health and Human Services. Summary of the HIPAA privacy rule. Available at: http://www.hhs.gov/ocr/privacy/hipaa/understanding/summary/index.html. Accessed October 9, 2012.

51. Data Protection Act 1998. Available at: http://www.legislation.gov.uk/ukpga/1998/29/section/2. Accessed October 12, 2012.

52. Eichler HG, Abadie E, Breckenridge A, et al. Open clinical trial data for all? A view from regulators. PLoS Med 2012;9:e1001202. Available at: http://www.plosmedicine.org/article/info%3Adoi%2F10.1371%2Fjournal.pmed.1001202. Accessed October 25, 2012.

53. Gliklich RE, Dreyer NA, editors. Registries for evaluating patient outcomes: a user's guide. 2nd edition. Rockville (MD): Agency for Healthcare Research and Quality; 2010. Available at: http://effectivehealthcare.ahrq.gov/index.cfm/search-for-guides-reviews-and-reports/?pageaction=display product&productID=531; 2010. Accessed October 25, 2012.

54. Weitzman ER, Kaci L, Mandl KD. Sharing medical data for health research: the early personal health record experience. J Med Internet Res 2010;12: e14. Available at: http://www.jmir.org/2010/2/e14/. Accessed October 25, 2012.

55. Weitzman ER, Kelemen S, Kaci L, et al. Willingness to share personal health record data for care improvement and public health: a survey of

experienced personal health record users. BMC Med Inform Decis Mak 2012;12:39. Available at: http://www.biomedcentral.com/1472-6947/12/39. Accessed October 25, 2012.

56. Joober R, Schmitz N, Annable L, et al. Publication bias: what are the challenges and can they be overcome? J Psychiatry Neurosci 2012;37: 149–52.

57. Keyes GR, Singer R, Iverson RE, et al. Analysis of outpatient surgery center safety using an internet-based quality improvement and peer review program. Plast Reconstr Surg 2004;113: 1760–70.

58. Keyes GR, Singer R, Iverson RE, et al. Mortality in outpatient surgery. Plast Reconstr Surg 2008;122: 245–50.

Outpatient Surgery and Sequelae
An Analysis of the AAAASF Internet-based Quality Assurance and Peer Review Database

Ali M. Soltani, MD[a], Geoffrey R. Keyes, MD[b,c],*,
Robert Singer, MD[d,e], Lawrence Reed, MD[f],
Peter B. Fodor, MD[g]

KEYWORDS

- Plastic and reconstructive surgery • Outpatient surgery • Sequelae

KEY POINTS

- The Internet-based quality assurance and Peer Review Program (IBQAP) has demonstrated the safety of procedures performed in the outpatient setting through the analysis of outcomes, the future of patient care will be directed by evidence-based medicine.
- Large inpatient surgical databases, such as the National Surgical Quality Improvement Program, the Nationwide Inpatient Sample, and the National Trauma Database, have long existed to provide quality assurance and improvement data for the inpatient cohort of patients.
- The acquisition of large data sets related to surgical care can best be achieved through the Internet.
- However, the structure of the data points must encompass the entire care process, from preoperative preparation to postoperative management.
- When outcomes are analyzed in conjunction with the indications for a procedure and the manner that care was delivered, evidence-based medicine is the end product.

INTRODUCTION

The number of surgical procedures performed in outpatient surgery facilities has increased dramatically over the past 20 years as a result of the development of safe standards for operation.[1,2] According to the National Center for Health Statistics, outpatient procedures performed in community hospitals in the United States increased from 16% in 1980 to 63% in 2005.[3] The growth of free-standing and office-based ambulatory surgery facilities has exceeded the number of hospital-based facilities. However, legislation requiring accreditation or licensure of these facilities has been slow to evolve. At this time, half of the states do not require any oversight of outpatient facilities.

The specialty of Plastic and Reconstructive surgery has been instrumental in supporting accreditation and licensure for outpatient surgery. Founded by Plastic Surgeons, the American Association for Accreditation of Ambulatory Surgery

[a] Division of Plastic, Reconstructive and Aesthetic Surgery, University of Miami/Jackson Memorial Hospital, Miami, Florida; [b] American Association for Accreditation of Ambulatory Surgery Facilities, Inc (AAAASF), Gurnee, Illinois, USA; [c] Department of Plastic Surgery, Keck School of Medicine, University of Southern California, Los Angeles, California; [d] University of California, San Diego, CA, USA; [e] American Association for Accreditation of Ambulatory Surgery Facilities, Inc (AAAASF), La Jolla, California; [f] The Weill Cornell Medical Center, New York Presbyterian Hospital, New York, USA; [g] UCLA Medical Center, Los Angeles, California, USA
* Corresponding author.
E-mail address: geoffreykeyes@sbcglobal.net

Clin Plastic Surg 40 (2013) 465–473
http://dx.doi.org/10.1016/j.cps.2013.04.010

Facilities (AAAASF), Inc was established in 1980 to develop an accreditation program to standardize and improve the quality of medical and surgical care in ambulatory surgery facilities while assuring the public of high standards for patient care and safety in an accredited facility. AAAASF now accredits single-specialty and multispecialty facilities accounting for most surgical specialties, including gastroenterology, podiatry, and oral and maxillofacial surgery. As the largest organization in the country that accredits office-based surgery centers, AAAASF has been engaged in the movement to mandate accreditation or licensure of outpatient surgery facilities nationally. AAAASF's main focus is safety and the improvement of patient care.[4,5]

In 1995 AAAASF championed AB 595 (Speier) in California that mandated accreditation or licensure for outpatient facilities in that state. In 2001 the American Society of Plastic Surgeons and the American Society for Aesthetic Plastic Surgery took a strong position in the effort to improve patient safety by mandating that their members operate only in accredited or licensed facilities.[4,5]

All surgical specialties now routinely perform some of their procedures on an outpatient basis. The outpatient surgery setting offers convenience, patient privacy and comfort, increased efficiency, and lower costs.

Those facilities that are accredited or licensed by the state, either free standing or office based, must comply with recognized standards of operation to safeguard patient care. Monitoring compliance with these standards is vital to ensure patient safety.

With this concept in mind, AAAASF, now the largest organization in the United States that accredits single-specialty or multispecialty office-based surgery centers, has taken the lead in evaluating compliance with standards through monitoring outcomes in their facilities. A major advance in this process was the development of the first Internet-based quality assurance database program (IBQAP).[6]

In recent years there have been numerous inpatient databases used to monitor surgical and medical outcomes, but there were no national databases providing an overview of outcomes in the outpatient arena. IBQAP was created in 1999 to fill that void.[6]

DATA COLLECTION

AAAASF standards require all accredited facilities to institute an ongoing quality improvement program that monitors and evaluates the quality of patient care, creates methods to improve patient care, and identifies and corrects deficiencies within their facilities. In adhering to this standard, all surgeons in accredited facilities must enter random case reports and all unanticipated sequelae into IBQAP. Peer review must be performed every 6 months. If peer review sources external to the facility are used to evaluate delivery of surgical care, the patient consent form is written to protect the confidentiality of the medical records, consistent with current HIPAA and other legal standards.

PEER REVIEW

Peer review is performed either by a recognized peer review organization or by a physician other than the operating surgeon. A minimum of 6 random cases per surgeon using the facility must be reviewed, and for group practices, 2% of all cases performed. These random case reviews must include assessment of the following 7 items:

1. Thoroughness and legibility of the history and physical examination
2. Adequacy and appropriateness of the surgical consent form
3. Presence of appropriate laboratory, electrocardiographic, and radiographic reports
4. Presence of a dictated operative report or its equivalent
5. Anesthesia record for operations performed with intravenous sedation or general anesthesia
6. Presence of instructions for postoperative and follow-up care
7. Documentation of unanticipated sequelae.

All unanticipated operative sequelae must be entered, including, but not limited to, the following 9 defined categories:

1. Unplanned hospital admission
2. Unscheduled return to the operating room for complication of a previous procedure
3. Untoward complications of a procedure, such as infection, bleeding, wound dehiscence, or inadvertent injury to another body structure
4. Cardiac or respiratory problems during stay at the facility or within 48 hours of discharge
5. Allergic reaction to medication
6. Incorrect needle or sponge count
7. Patient or family complaint
8. Equipment malfunction leading to injury or potential injury to patient
9. Death

Each unanticipated operative sequela chart review includes the following 5 informational items, in addition to the operative procedure performed:

1. Identification of the problem
2. Immediate treatment or disposition of the case

3. Outcome
4. Analysis of reason for problem
5. Assessment of efficacy of treatment.

Morbidity and mortality data are entered and analyzed through the AAAASF mandated peer review program. Keyes and colleagues[6] first reported on outcomes data from the IBQAP system in 2004, recommending expansion of the range and scope of the collection process to enhance analysis further. Another article published in 2008 reported the incidence of deaths after outpatient surgery.[7]

ANALYSIS OF SEQUELAE
Overview

AAAASF has grown dramatically in the past 10 years and now accredits surgeons from all surgical specialties, gastroenterology, oral and maxillofacial surgery, and podiatry. For this review, an analysis of outcomes on all procedures performed in AAAASF accredited facilities from 2001 through 2012 was conducted. There were a total of 7,629,686 procedures performed on 5,416,071 patients. Procedures performed by specialties other than plastic surgery are excluded from this study. There were 5,525,225 plastic surgery procedures performed on 3,922,202 patients. The average number of procedures performed per patient was 1.41.

There were 21,994 sequelae reported. The overall incidence of sequelae in all plastic surgery procedures was 0.40% or 1 in 251 procedures and, for cases, 0.56% or 1 in 178 cases. The average of procedures per case was 1.41.

The 5 most common surgical procedures performed were breast augmentation, abdominoplasty, mastopexy/reduction mammoplasty, liposuction, and facelift and related procedures (**Fig. 1**).

Abdominoplasty was the procedure most commonly associated with a sequela. The overall incidence of unanticipated sequelae with abdominoplasty was 0.925%. A comparison of sequelae rates for the top 5 procedures performed is shown in **Fig. 2**.

SEQUELAE TYPES
Hematoma

Postoperative bleeding or hematoma was by far the most common complication (**Fig. 3**). There were 7931 hematomas, more than twice the number of infections in the reported time period. **Fig. 4** shows the top 5 procedures and their number of hematomas. There were 535 patients hospitalized because of a hematoma, which is an incidence of 0.20% for all plastic surgery cases performed. Of hematomas, 6.75% were hospitalized. There were no deaths that occurred as a result of bleeding or hematoma. The increasing

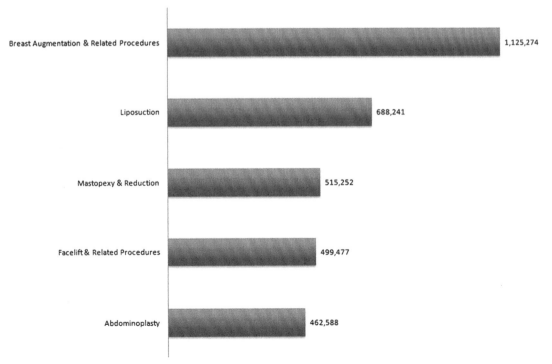

Fig. 1. Top 5 surgical procedures.

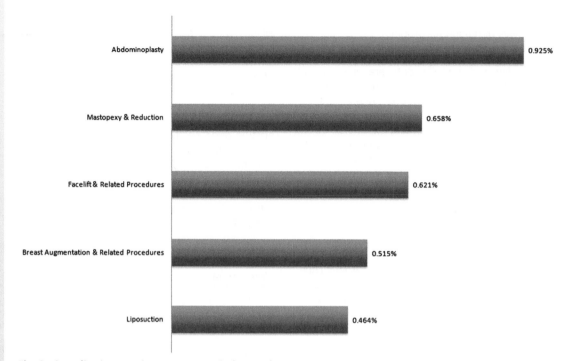

Fig. 2. Complication rate in common surgical procedures.

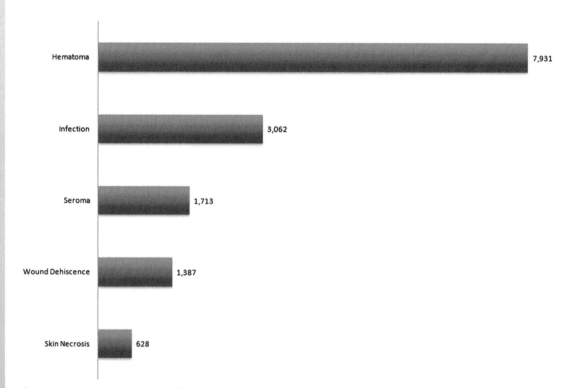

Fig. 3. Top 5 most common complications.

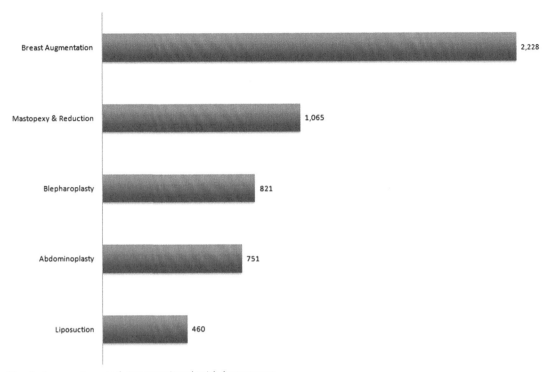

Fig. 4. Frequent procedures associated with hematoma.

awareness of the need for chemoprophylaxis to prevent the occurrence of venous thromboembolism (VTE) makes it likely that some of these patients received anticoagulation postoperatively. These data do not include information on chemoprophylaxis, but the updated IBQAP database will monitor this issue to determine incidence of bleeding as a result of its use.

Infection

There were 3063 infections reported for the 3,922,202 cases performed. Infections were a rare complication with an incidence of 0.08% of all cases and 0.06% of procedures. Infection accounted for 14% of all sequelae. Infections were identified in 921 breast augmentations, 757 abdominoplasties, 582 mastopexies or related procedures, 517 liposuctions, and 346 facelifts or related procedures. The percentage of infections with specific procedures is shown in **Fig. 5**. The most common organisms cultured were *Staphylococcus aureus*, both methicillin-sensitive and methicillin-resistant, and *Serratia marcescens*. A more detailed report of infections in outpatient surgery is covered in another article in this volume.

Venous Thromboembolism

VTE, deep venous thrombi (DVT), and pulmonary emboli (PE) are serious sequelae that occur in procedures performed in either an inpatient or an outpatient surgery setting. There were 479 incidences of VTE including 215 DVTs and 264 PEs, an incidence of 0.012% or 1 in 8188 cases. Of the 264 PEs, 40 were fatal, representing a mortality rate of 15%.

There were 462,564 abdominoplasties performed in AAAASF facilities during the period reviewed. Approximately two-thirds of the time an abdominoplasty was combined with other surgical procedures. Combining abdominoplasty with 1 or 2 other procedures increased the risk of VTE and specifically PE. However, when abdominoplasty was combined with 3 procedures, the incidence did not increase. There were far fewer cases of abdominoplasty performed with 3 other procedures.

Figs. 6 and **7** illustrate the incidence of VTE and PE occurring when an abdominoplasty was performed alone or in combination with other procedures. The occurrence of VTE in any abdominoplasty procedure was 0.066% or 1 in 1502. That compares to the overall risk of VTE in all plastic surgical procedures of 0.012%, or 1 in 8188. That equals an odds ratio of approximately 5.5 (95% CI 4.7–6.3) and a P value of <0.001 using χ^2 analysis. All analyses were performed using STATA version 12 software (Stata Corp, College Station, TX, USA). Abdominoplasty is a procedure that has an increased risk of VTE, including both DVT and PE.

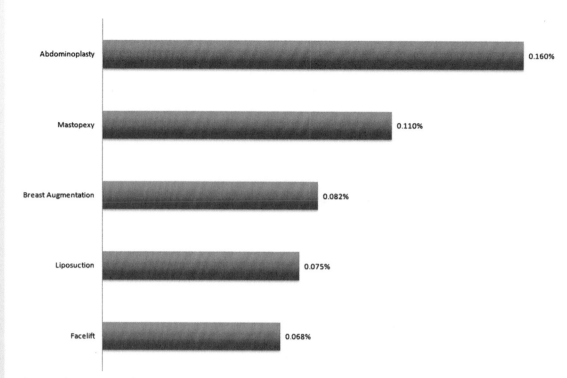

Fig. 5. Infection Rate of most common procedures.

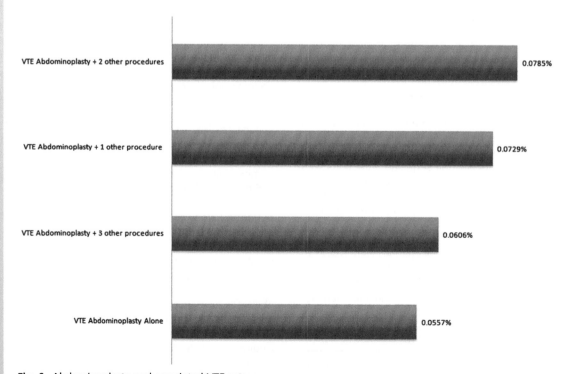

Fig. 6. Abdominoplasty and associated VTE rates.

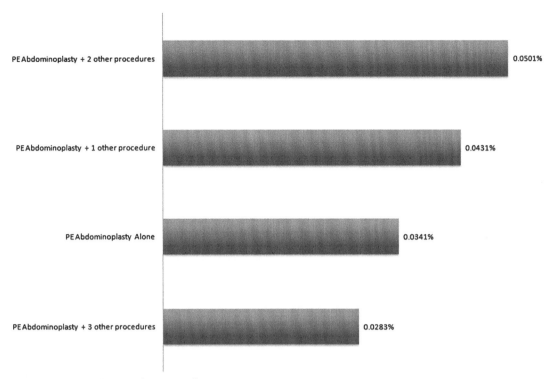

Fig. 7. Abdominoplasty and associated PE rates.

Pneumothorax

Pneumothorax, an uncommon sequela, occurred in 120 cases, an incidence of 0.0031%. Seventy-seven or one-half of the reported pneumothoraces occurred with breast augmentations. Detailed information on the breakdown of the occurrence of pneumothoraces by procedures can be found in **Fig. 8**.

Mortality

There were 94 deaths occurring between 2001 and 2012. Mortality is a rare occurrence in outpatient surgery, with an incidence of 0.0017% of all procedures or 0.0024% of total cases. The risk of death for a patient having any plastic surgery was approximately 1 in 41,726.

PE was by far the most common cause of death, with 40 cases of PE causing mortality. Of these 40 deaths, 26 were associated with abdominoplasty. Most fatal PEs, 20, were in cases where abdominoplasty was combined with other procedures. PE was previously reported as the leading cause of death in outpatient surgery in prior reports.[7] Other causes of mortality were cardiac arrhythmia, myocardial infarction, and drug overdose. **Fig. 9** lists the causes of death within the study population.

DISCUSSION

Hematomas or postoperative bleeding was the most common complication occurring in patients evaluated in this study. Bleeding was most frequently associated with breast augmentation.

Although mortality in an outpatient facility is a relatively rare occurrence, an understanding of what care interventions are necessary to reduce its incidence will come through improved data analysis. As previously reported, the most common cause of death was a PE, which in many instances is a preventable event. Numerous patient safety articles have been published describing preoperative evaluation for the prevention of pulmonary embolism using chemoprophylaxis.[8–12] Abdominoplasty is the procedure associated with the highest rate of sequelae and specifically VTE. In this study, abdominoplasty was the most frequently implicated surgery in patients with fatal PE. Abdominoplasty is associated with a 5.5 times greater risk for the development of VTE than any other plastic surgical procedures.

IBQAP data on VTE have led to the development of a new standard by AAAASF mandating documentation of the preoperative clinical evaluation of patients at risk for a VTE. This screening may be performed using the Caprini Evaluation Tool, guidelines set forth by the American College of

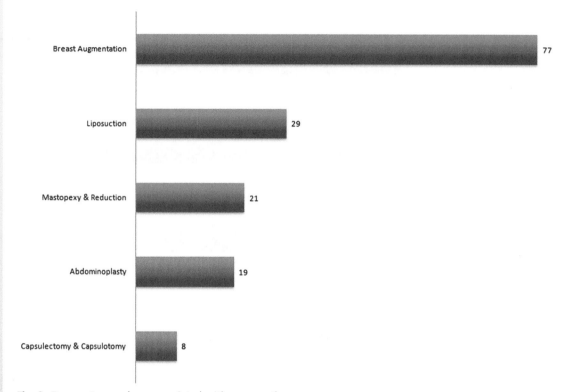

Fig. 8. Frequent procedures associated with pneumothorax.

Chest Physicians, or other comparable assessment guidelines.[12]

Pneumothorax, while exceeding rare, at approximately 0.0031% of cases, is a sequela that requires immediate attention in the operating room. Most of these cases were in patients having breast augmentation. Outpatient surgery facilities should be equipped to manage this complication.

Sporadic reports in the news about infections in outpatient surgery have raised the question about its frequency in the outpatient setting. In AAAASF accredited facilities, the incidence of infection is low. It is important to remember that not all infections begin in the surgery facility environment. Proper postoperative wound care is of the utmost importance in the postoperative environment.

SUMMARY

Although Internet-based quality assurance and peer review data have demonstrated the safety of procedures performed in the outpatient setting through the analysis of outcomes, the future of patient care will be directed by evidence-based medicine. Large inpatient surgical databases, such as the National Surgical Quality Improvement Program, the Nationwide Inpatient Sample, and the National Trauma Database, have long existed to provide quality assurance and improvement data for the inpatient cohort of patients.[13] Internet-based quality assurance and peer review has led the way in the collection of data for outpatient surgery facilities.

The acquisition of large data sets related to surgical care can best be achieved through the Internet. However, the structure of the data points

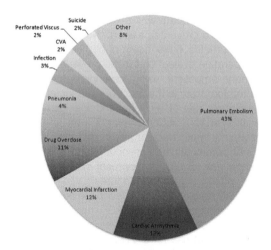

Fig. 9. Causes of death. CVA, cerebrovascular accident. CVA, cerebrovascular accident.

must encompass the entire care process, from preoperative preparation to postoperative management. When outcomes are analyzed in conjunction with the indications for a procedure and the manner that care was delivered, evidence-based medicine is the end product. An example of this concept is the knowledge that chemoprophylaxis was or was not used in a procedure whose outcome resulted in the development of a VTE. The data collected in the AAAASF peer review system document the safety of outpatient surgery in their facilities, but there is room for improvement. The new system will have the ability to digitalize important aspects of the entire care process to enhance the value of the data. Centralization of data collection through the Internet from the multiple accrediting, licensing, and patient care managing entities will provides the means of assessing the surgical process to achieve this goal, which will evolve through the development of a data hub.

REFERENCES

1. Rohrich RJ, White PF. Safety of outpatient surgery: is mandatory accreditation of outpatient surgery centers enough? Plast Reconstr Surg 2001;107:189.

2. Byrd HS, Barton FE, Orenstein HH, et al. Safety and efficacy in an accredited outpatient plastic surgery facility: a review of 5316 consecutive cases. Plast Reconstr Surg 2003;112:636.

3. Haeck PC, Swanson JA, Iverson RE, et al. Evidence-based patient safety advisory: patient selection and procedures in ambulatory surgery. Plast Reconstr Surg 2009;124(Suppl 4):6S–27S.

4. Iverson RA, Lynch DJ, the ASPS Task Force on Patient Safety in Office-Based Surgery Facilities. Patient safety in office-based facilities: II. Patient selection. Plast Reconstr Surg 2002;110:1785.

5. American Association for Accreditation of Ambulatory Surgical Facilities, Inc. AAAASF Standards and Checklist for Accreditation of Ambulatory Surgery Facilities. Mundelein (IL): American Association for Accreditation of Ambulatory Surgical Facilities; 1999.

6. Keyes GR, Singer R, Iverson RE, et al. Analysis of outpatient surgery center safety using an internet-based quality improvement and peer review program. Plast Reconstr Surg 2004;113(6):1760–70.

7. Keyes GR, Singer R, Iverson RE, et al. Mortality in outpatient surgery. Plast Reconstr Surg 2008;122(1):245–50 [discussion: 251–3].

8. Hoefflin SM, Bornstein JB, Gordon M. General anesthesia in an office-based plastic surgery facility: a report on more than 23,000 consecutive office based procedures under general anesthesia with no significant anesthetic complications. Plast Reconstr Surg 2001;107:243.

9. Singer R. General anesthesia in an office-based surgical facility: a report on more than 23,000 consecutive office-based procedures under general anesthesia with no significant anesthetic complications. Plast Reconstr Surg 2001;107:252 [discussion].

10. American Society of Plastic Surgeons and American Society for Aesthetic Plastic Surgery. Policy statement on accreditation of office facilities. Arlington (VA): American Society of Plastic Surgeons; Available at: http://www.plasticsurgery.org/psf/psfhome/govern/officepol.cfm. Accessed October 22, 2012.

11. Morello DC, Colon GA, Fredricks S, et al. Patient safety in accredited office surgical facilities. Plast Reconstr Surg 1997;96:1496.

12. Pannucci CJ, Bailey SH, Dreszer G, et al. Validation of the Caprini risk assessment model in plastic and reconstructive surgery patients. J Am Coll Surg 2011;212(1):105–12.

13. Reinke CE, Karakousis GC, Hadler RA, et al. Incidence of venous thromboembolism in patients undergoing surgical treatment for malignancy by type of neoplasm: an analysis of ACS-NSQIP data from 2005 to 2010. Surgery 2012;152(2):186–92.

Preventing Surgical Mishaps
Using Surgical Checklists

John D. Newkirk, PhD, MD

KEYWORDS

- Surgery • Checklist • Complications • Mortality • Morbidity

KEY POINTS

- Surgical checklists decreases complications and saves lives.
- The use of a checklist improves surgical culture.

BACKGROUND: CHECKLISTS STARTED IN THE AERONAUTIC INDUSTRY

In the summer of 1934, the US Army Air Corps circulated a proposal for a new long-range bomber to replace the 2-engined B-10, which was currently in use. Prospective builders were instructed to have multiengined aircraft ready for a competition in October 1935. The candidate aircraft had to be able to fly at least 1640 km (1020 miles) and preferably 3540 km (2200 miles). They had to be able to carry a 900-kg (2000-pound) bomb load and to be able to reach a speed of at least 320 kph (200 mph), although 400 kph (250 mph) was considered desirable.

Working in secrecy, Boeing produced a prototype, the Model 299. When a Seattle newspaperman saw the prototype, he named it a "flying fortress"; the name stuck. The Model 299 had 4 engines, rather than 2 or 3; retractable landing gear; electric trim tabs on its control surfaces; a hydraulically operated constant-speed propeller; and positions on the fuselage for gun turrets. It was a more complicated plane than the B-10 and was the first 4-engined plane ever built.

After a short period of testing the 299 was delivered to Wright Field, Ohio, for testing against a Martin design, an upgraded B-10, and a DC-2 Douglas converted into a bomber, the DB-1. Both were good designs, but were 2-engined aircraft. Boeing's 299 Flying Fortress was in a class by itself. It could carry 5 tons of bombs, depending on the fuel load, which was far more than its 2-engined competitors; the 299 carried its load higher, faster, and nearly twice as far as its competitors.

On October 30, 1935, the Fortress prototype taxied out for takeoff at Wright Field. A crowd gathered to watch. At the controls was the Air Corps' chief test pilot, Major Ployer P. Hill. His copilot was First Lt. Donald L. Putt. Also aboard were an engineer, a mechanic (both were in the rear) and Leslie R. Tower, the Boeing test pilot, who was standing in the cockpit behind the two pilots.

The aircraft roared down the runway and took off. It then climbed steeply-too steeply. It rose to an altitude of about 90 m (300 ft), where it stalled, rolled to the side, crashed back onto the airfield and exploded. Putt and Tower stumbled out of the wreckage dazed and bleeding. The two mechanics went out the back, largely unscathed. Hill was unconscious and trapped in the cockpit. He was evacuated from the wreckage but died the next day. Tower, who had been standing behind the pilots as an observer, blamed himself for the accident. Although he did not seem to be seriously injured, he died not long afterward.

Investigators determined that the Fortress crashed because the elevator and rudder controls

Funding Source: None.
Conflict of Interest: None.
Private Practice, 3020 Sunset Boulevard, Suite 100, West Columbia, Columbia, SC 29169-3494, USA
E-mail address: jdn@columbiaplasticsurgery.com

Clin Plastic Surg 40 (2013) 475–487
http://dx.doi.org/10.1016/j.cps.2013.04.011
0094-1298/13/$ – see front matter © 2013 Elsevier Inc. All rights reserved.

were locked; the pilot could not lower the nose, so the aircraft quickly stalled. The locking mechanism was controlled from inside the cockpit, but no one remembered to disengage it before takeoff. Tower apparently noticed that the control lock was still engaged as the aircraft moved up to stall, but was unable to get to it in time to prevent a crash. More familiar with the 299 than anyone else, this oversight on his part is why he blamed himself for the disaster. Because the Boeing prototype had crashed, the Corps declared the winner to be the Douglas DB-1, later designated the B-18 Bolo.

Air Corps leaders tried to place an order for 65 of the revolutionary Fortresses, but War Department General Staff, who controlled Air Corps finances, refused. The General Staff advanced the view that, because the Boeing airplane had crashed, it must have been too complex for anyone to handle safely. Acting on the misguided principle that quantity was more important than quality, the Army promptly ordered 133 of the new Bolos.

A group of test pilots thought that the Flying Fortress, although complex, was flyable. They came up with a checklist for pilots to use before take off, while taxiing, during flight, and landing, to ensure that some simple but crucial step, such as unlocking the elevator and rudder controls, had not been forgotten. Through a legal loophole, the Air Corps was eventually able to purchase 13 Flying Fortresses, enough to equip 1 squadron. These planes were designated YB-17s. Using the checklists, Air Corps pilots logged more than 9200 flying hours on their YB-17s without experiencing a serious major accident.

When World War II broke out in Europe in September 1939, the Army Air Corps had barely 24 of the new B-17s. In September 1940, the number was up to only 49 bombers. The United States needed to increase production, but things still moved at a glacial pace. At the time of Japan's attack on Pearl Harbor on December 7, 1941, the Air Corps had fewer than 200 B-17s in the inventory. Not until early 1944 would the US military have enough Fortresses to have a decisive impact on the bombing campaign against Germany. The Army eventually purchased about 13,000 Flying Fortresses. Three-hundred and fifty Bolos were purchased. They proved unsatisfactory in combat and were relegated to coastal patrols and navigational training.

The 1935 crash did produce one notable benefit. Airmen realized that aircraft were becoming too complex to fly safely without standardized procedures. Moreover, these procedures were too numerous and complicated to commit entirely to memory. Checklists were developed that spelled out specific tasks that were to be accomplished by each crew member at various times throughout the flight and also while on the ground. Such a checklist, performed while taxiing out for takeoff, would probably have revealed that the 299's elevator locks were still engaged. Today, such detailed checklists are mandatory for all aircraft.[1]

LESSONS OF THE AERONAUTIC INDUSTRY EXTENDED TO HEALTH CARE: A CHECKLIST AND BLOODSTREAM INFECTIONS

It may seem strange to try to adapt techniques devised to make flying complicated aircraft safe to the practice of medicine, but, in 2001, a physician at Johns Hopkins Hospital, Peter Pronovost, PhD, MD, decided to try to put one together to decrease the rate of complications of one of the tasks that physicians do daily in most hospitals: placement of central lines.

In 2006 it was reported that 36 million patients were admitted to hospitals in the United States, staying for 164 million hospital days. Eleven percent of those hospital days are spent in intensive care units (ICUs), or 9.7 million days; for 54% of the days (9.7 million), central venous catheters remain in place to infuse medicine and fluids.[2] At that time there were 48,600 catheter-related bloodstream infections resulting in deaths estimated from 17,000[2] to 28,000 per year.[3] The median rate of catheter-related bloodstream infections in ICUs ranged from 1.8 to 5.2 per 1000 catheter days.[4]

The intervention used evidence-based procedures recommended by the Communicable Disease Center as having the greatest effect on decreasing the rate of catheter-related bloodstream infection. These procedures were that physicians wash their hands before the catheter placement; full barrier protection is placed on the patient before insertion of the catheter; the physician wears sterile gloves, mask, hat and gown; the skin of the patient is scrubbed with chlorhexidine; the femoral site should be avoided, if possible; and unnecessary catheters should be removed as soon as possible. Dr Pronovost devised a 1-page checklist to ensure that these tasks were performed. Nurses stopped providers in nonemergency situations from proceeding with catheter placement if the steps were not followed.

This checklist was tried out at Johns Hopkins Hospital; results were dramatic: the 10-day infection rate went from 11% to 0%. Pronovost then devised checklists to ensure that nurses observed patients for pain at least once every 4 hours, which reduced the likelihood of patients enduring pain from 41% to 3%. Another checklist ensured that patients on mechanical ventilators received antacid medication and that the head of the bed was propped up to at least 30°.

The percentage of patients not receiving antacids went from 70% to 4%; the incidence of pneumonia decreased about 25%. Checklists helped with memory recall, established the minimum necessary steps in a process, and established a higher standard of baseline performance.[5,6]

The checklist to reduce catheter-induced infections was introduced in most of the ICUs in Michigan as part of a statewide safety initiative known as the Michigan Health and Hospital Association (MHA) Patient Safety and Quality Keystone Center ICU project. The project also introduced a daily goals sheet to improve clinician-to-clinician communication within the ICU, an intervention to reduce ventilator-assisted pneumonia, and a comprehensive unit-based safety program to improve safety culture. The project involved 67 hospitals, of which 52% were teaching facilities and included 85% of all of the ICU beds in Michigan.[3]

Data were collected from 103 ICUs for 1981 ICU months and 375,757 catheter days. Using the checklists, the overall median rate of catheter-related bloodstream infection decreased from 2.7 (mean 7.7) infections per 1000 catheter days at baseline to 0 (mean 2.3) at 0 to 3 months after implementation of the study intervention, and was sustained at 0 (mean 1.4) during 18 months of follow-up. Teaching and nonteaching hospitals realized similar improvements.[3]

These data were published in the *New England Journal of Medicine*. An editorial in the same issue discussing this article stated that "the story is compelling and the costs and efforts so relatively minor that the five components of the intervention should be widely adopted. We can no longer accept the variations in safety culture, behavior or systems of practice that have plagued medical care for decades. Imagine the effect if all 6000 acute care hospitals in the United States were to show a similar commitment and discipline."[2]

DEVELOPMENT OF THE WORLD HEALTH ORGANIZATION CHECKLIST

In an article published in 2008, Weiser and colleagues,[7] reported that the World Health Organization (WHO) had collected demographic, economic, and health data from the 192 WHO member states. WHO estimated that 232 million major surgical procedures are performed each year. The article concluded that "Worldwide volume of surgery is large. In view of the high death and complication rates of major surgical procedures, surgical safety should now be a substantial global public-health concern. The disproportionate scarcity of surgical access in low-income settings suggests a large unaddressed disease burden worldwide. Public-health efforts and surveillance in surgery should be established."

In January 2007 in Geneva, Switzerland, the first meeting of Safe Surgery Saves Lives convened for a 2-day conference, bringing together surgeons, anesthesiologists, nurses, hospital administrators, and others to improve the safety of surgery worldwide and to obtain better information on the nature of surgical services in different countries and in different health systems.

The group concluded that a surgical checklist should be developed. The checklist should ensure that proper antibiotics were given before incising the skin and that monitored anesthesia was administered. The checklist would emphasize teamwork and be occupied with measures that promote safety. It should include a preoperative briefing to address surgical team issues and also be a team training process. The checklist should facilitate teamwork. Members at the conference in Geneva recognized that different countries and different specialties would have different needs; the checklist should therefore provide latitude for additions and tailoring based on local factors and environment.[7] The checklist that was developed as a product of this conference and working sessions that followed is available at www.safesurgery.org and www.who.int/patientsafety/safe surgery/tools.

The WHO checklist contained 19 items to be noted before and after surgery: that patients confirmed their identity, surgical site, and procedure, and that a consent was signed; if applicable, the surgical site was marked; a pulse oximeter was present and functioning; members of the team were aware if the patient had a drug allergy; airway had been evaluated; and, if blood loss of at least 500 mL was expected, blood and fluids were available.[8] The goal was to create a tool that supported clinical practice without substituting a rigid algorithm for professional judgment. Following the aviation lesson, the checklist was to focus on items that are recognized to either be deadly if missed or, if not deadly, then high risk and known to be recurrently overlooked or missed.[9]

In the WHO checklist, a time-out is performed before skin incision. The patient's name, surgical site, and procedure are reviewed. All team members are identified by name and role; surgical, anesthesia, and nursing staff review the anticipated events and confirm that preoperative antibiotics have been administered. All imaging studies for the correct patient are displayed in the operating room, if necessary. Following surgery, the nurse reviews the name of the procedure and that needle, sponge, and instrument counts were correct. Any specimen, if necessary, has been labeled. Issues with equipment are addressed.

Between October 2007 and September 2008 8 hospitals in 8 cities (Toronto, Canada; New Delhi, India; Amman, Jordan; Auckland, New Zealand; Manila, Philippines; Ifakara, Tanzania; London, United Kingdom; and Seattle, WA) participated in the WHO's Safe Surgery Saves Lives program. Selection of these cities purposely included places with different economic circumstances and different populations. The checklist was introduced into these hospitals, each of which had a full-time investigator for the project with no other clinical responsibilities. Each hospital identified 1 to 4 operating rooms to serve as study rooms. Patients who were 16 years of age or older and were undergoing noncardiac surgery were consecutively enrolled in the study. After noting the practices at that time in each institution, all were asked to correct policies not consistent with the 19-item WHO safe-surgery checklist and to implement the checklist in the designated rooms. Part of the data was collected by observers in the operating room and part by clinical teams involved in surgical care.

During the baseline period 3733 patients were enrolled; 3955 patients were enrolled after the checklist was implemented. The rate of complications decreased from 11% at baseline to 7% after the checklist was introduced. The total in-hospital rate of death decreased from 1.5% to 0.8%. These decreases were of about 36%. Similar declines in complications were observed in high-income and in low-income sites. It was noted that, "The rates of reduction in rates of death and complications suggest that the checklist program can improve the safety of surgical patients in diverse clinical and economic environments."[8]

There have been some legitimate questions raised about the findings of the 8-hospital WHO study. Martin and colleagues[10] thought that a 30% reduction in death was unlikely to be achieved in the United Kingdom because rates of death in some hospitals in the WHO exceeded the published normal range of 0.4% to 0.8%. McCambridge and colleagues[11] noted that clinical teams were aware that they were being observed and that some of the improved outcomes may have been influenced by alterations in behavior. Sanders and Jameson[12] thought it was possible that antibiotics and pulse oximetry may have accounted for the survival advantage in the sites in cities of low income. In response to these doubts, Haynes and Gwande[13] pointed out that the case mix varied widely among hospitals and that the

hospitals had enormous diversity. Rate of postoperative death is unknown for the mix of cases in this international group of hospitals and comparison of these hospitals with those in developed countries is invalid. WHO recommends that the use of an oximeter and antibiotics are minimum standards for safe surgery. Haynes and Gwande[13] found no effect of an observer in the operating rooms.

Many of the findings of the WHO Safe Surgery Saves Lives study were confirmed in a tertiary university hospital in Utrecht, the Netherlands.[14]

EXPERIENCE WITH CHECKLISTS IN THE US VETERANS HEALTH ADMINISTRATION

The US Veterans Health Administration (VHA) is the largest national integrated health care system in the United States, with 153 hospitals of which 130 provide surgical services. In 2006, the VHA implemented a team training program for operating room personnel on a national level that included 2 months of preparation, a 1-day conference, and 1 year of quarterly coaching interviews. It involved briefing and debriefing in the operating room and included checklists as an integral part of the process. Data were collected from 2006, 2007, and 2008, and compared mortality before and after team training and checklists were implemented. Baseline mortality for the 42 facilities that received training in 2007 was their 2006 rate; baseline mortality for the 32 that underwent training in 2008 was their 2007 rate. Thirty-four facilities did not receive training in those 3 years.

After controlling for variables, the 74 trained facilities observed an 18% reduction in mortality. For every quarter of training that the facilities received there was measurable decrease in mortality. The dose-response relationship between the training programs with inclusion of the control of the previous year's statistics supports the conclusion that training caused the reduction in mortality rather than other influences that may have occurred.[15]

DUTCH EXPERIENCE WITH THE SURGICAL PATIENT SAFETY SYSTEM CHECKLIST

In 2010, a Dutch group published results of a study to reduce complications in surgical patients.[16] Starting with the WHO checklist, the group developed the Surgical Patient Safety System (SURPASS) checklist. The pathway was subdivided into admission to the ward, operating room, recovery/ICU, ward, and discharge. This checklist was multidisciplinary: ward doctor, surgeon, anesthesiologist, operating room assistant, and nurses were responsible for completion of parts of the checklist.[17] The checklist was designed to provide a comprehensive pathway, minimize information loss during transfers from one stage of the pathway, and to promote interdisciplinary communication. The nearly 100 items on the checklist required that 11 forms be completed and documented.[18]

The checklist was used in 6 academic or tertiary teaching hospitals. Five academic or tertiary teaching hospitals were used as controls. Ninety percent of procedures observed in each group of hospitals were procedures that required surgical intervention in less than 24 hours, gastrointestinal procedures, trauma, vascular, renal or amputation surgery, abdominal wall procedures, breast surgery, and endocrine surgery. In a comparison of 3760 patients observed before implementation of the checklist with 3820 patients observed after implementation of the checklist, complications per 100 patients decreased from 27.3 to 16.7. The proportion of patients with 1 or more complications decreased from 15.4% to 10.2%. In-hospital mortality decreased from 1.5% to 0.8%. Outcomes did not change in the control hospitals.[16] Use of the checklist also optimized timing of antibiotic prophylaxis.[19]

The study from the Netherlands documented a positive relationship between checklist compliance and outcomes. Patients with incomplete checklists had more complications than those for whom checklists were completed. It is not clear whether similar benefits would have been realized with fewer items. The WHO study achieved similar reductions in morbidity and mortality with a simpler checklist focused on the operating room alone.[18]

THE CHECKLIST TRIAL IN SOUTH CAROLINA

Following the development of the WHO checklist, 2 members of the Safe Surgery Saves Lives program decided to implement checklists in a trial state in the United States. Atul Gwande, MD, MPH, is a general and endocrine surgeon at the Brigham and Women's Hospital in Boston. He is an associate professor at Harvard Medical School and the Harvard School of Public Health and leads the Safe Surgery Saves Lives program for the WHO. William Berry, MD, is a former cardiac surgeon and chief scientist for Safe Surgery Saves Lives. Dr Berry is a professor in the School of Public Health of Harvard University.

Dr Gwande and Dr Berry chose South Carolina as the first state to implement surgical checklists. South Carolina was chosen because it is a small state: it is 24th in population and 40th in size. The South Carolina Hospital Association (SCHA)

has a history of working closely with South Carolina hospitals and had successfully introduced several safety initiatives, including getting patients into a catheterization laboratory within 90 minutes of a myocardial infarction and the formation of rapid response teams. The association between the SCHA and the Harvard School of Public Health was announced on September 18, 2010.

All of the hospitals in South Carolina committed to putting the checklist into routine use in their operating rooms by the end of 2013. Successful implementation and proper use of the checklist is expected to save more than 500 lives per year in South Carolina. The experiences of South Carolina hospitals will serve as a model to improve patient safety and change the face of surgery across the United States. The program is named safesurgery2015 (www.safesurgery2015.org).[20]

There are about 400,000 inpatient operations per year in South Carolina and about 60,000 outpatient surgical procedures. The program started in South Carolina involved 60 of 65 hospitals in the state. The checklist was not introduced to all 60 hospitals at once. The first wave included 23 hospitals and ran from April to November 2011. The second wave ran from November 2011 to April 2012 and the third wave targeted 29 hospitals and ran from April to October 2012. The goal was to decrease the death rate to less than 1%, which would be lower than the death rate in any state. The first year involved more than 1300 people, 140,000 hours of work, and 1600 hours of webinars and telecommunication. People in the program traveled 2400 miles in state and the CEOs of all of the hospitals were involved.[21]

Greenville Hospital System University Medical Center is a research institution nationally known for advanced technology and comprehensive services and staff. It is one of the largest health systems in the southeast and the largest in South Carolina. It is the only academic medical center in the upstate area with 746 beds. Greenville Memorial Hospital is the state's largest acute care hospital.

Christopher Wright, MD, is a cardiovascular surgeon in the Greenville Hospital System and is one of the physician champions in introducing the checklist to South Carolina. I interviewed him in Greenville and again at the SCHA meeting on October 17, 2012. The interviews indicate some of the practical problems in implementing the checklist statewide.

> Newkirk: "What is the background of the checklist in South Carolina?"
> Wright: "What we decided to do in Safe Surgery 2015 was to see if we could get a safety

checklist based on the WHO checklist in every hospital and every operating room by 2014. Dr Gwandi and Dr Berry introduced the idea about 3 years ago to get people on board. Thereafter we put together a leadership team of Dr Berry and myself. Dr Barry and his team [at the Harvard School of Public Health] did most of the process thinking and gave it to us to run with it. They asked me to go back to my hospital and set up a leadership team. That team took the World Health Organization checklist and used it or modified it, based on the hospital's needs. We also had webinars weekly. Anyone involved could view those webinars and have weekly office calls [to Harvard School of Public Health]. Dr Berry has the results to the surveys that were taken which included, 'Would you want to be operated in this operating room?' Dr Berry has the results to these surveys."

Newkirk: "What is the present situation in introducing the checklist in South Carolina?"

Wright: "We have some work to do on some smaller hospitals that are not on board. The biggest problem is getting people to use it and total commitment from the leadership. We are part of a project now to collect data to make sure the checklist is being used properly. We want to find a tool to measure that the checklist is being used appropriately.

We are using the same checklist in general surgery and cardiac surgery. We are looking to make different checklists, but the basic checklist will still be there.

I think communication within the health care system is crucial. One thing that I have learned is 75% of errors are committed by people, meaning only 25% of error is by the process. Most of the errors committed by people are based on a breakdown of communication. If we have any tool that can help communication among team members it will help and the check list will certainly do that. We don't really call it the checklist anymore we call it the 'surgery briefing and debriefing.' We are actively trying to get the mindset [in this hospital] that this isn't a checklist; this is a tool to make sure that all resources and information are at the point of care and that everyone in the room is communicating with each other. We need to be able to communicate on an equal basis and the checklist will allow is to do that. Each person has a role and by acknowledging that, it gets people communicating and talking. It makes people feel that they can talk and speak up. I have given the staff [in this hospital] the ability to speak out. When you announce who you are and what your role is at the beginning of an operation, you are more likely to speak up if you see a problem because you have already spoken up. What goes hand in hand with this is you have to develop an adjusted culture and what I mean by that is if someone speaks up and they are wrong you need to guide them instead of biting their head off. The checklist helps foster this idea and puts people on an equal basis."

Newkirk: "Have the physicians been amenable to the introduction of the checklist?"

Wright: "For the most part, yes. At least 90% of the doctors here are on board. I think what you really need is a couple of strong physician leaders who really believe in it to lead this project. Done right and done correctly it is well worth the time. Once you use it for a significant amount of time you will begin to change the culture in the room and [eventually] in health care globally. We are excited about it though we know there is a still a lot of work to be done. Not only does it make the one case safer, it is a vehicle for the institution as a whole to go toward quality improvement and communication improvement.

Newkirk: "How much of the WHO checklist did you change or modify?"

Wright: "Not too much. We made a surgeon component, nurse component, and an anesthesiologist component. For example, we do not dictate how every physician in the hospital does it. As long as you hit all the key points of the checklist the process does not matter. The key is that everyone introduces themselves and has the opportunity to speak up. Debriefing occurs at the end.

Newkirk: Tell me about the debriefing.

Wright: "Debriefing occurs at the end of the case. I will say 'does anyone have any concerns about this case?' If there are no concerns at the time the case is over. But if there are concerns we address them. Everything is discussed at the debriefing such as equipment problems or concerns about the patients that need to be documented for the next team taking over. We want our staff to function like a NASCAR pit crew. The checklist is one of those tools that can make

Before Induction of Anesthesia

Nurse and Anesthesia Provider review:
- ❑ Patient identification (name and DOB)
- ❑ Surgical site
- ❑ Surgical Procedure to be performed matches the consent
- ❑ The site has been marked
- ❑ Known allergies
- ❑ The anesthesia safety check has been completed

Anesthesia Provider discusses patient specific information with the team:
- ❑ **Anticipated airway or aspiration risk**
- ❑ **Risk of significant blood loss**
  - Two IVs/central access and fluids planned
  - Type and crossmatch/screen
  - Blood availability
- ❑ **Risk of hypothermia - operation >1h**
  - Warmer in place
- ❑ **Risk of venous thromboembolism**
  - Boots and/or anticoagulants in place

Before Skin Incision

Surgeon, Nurse, and Anesthesia Provider perform the Time Out:
- ❑ Patient's name
- ❑ Surgical procedure to be performed
- ❑ Surgical site
- ❑ Patient Positioning
- ❑ Essential imaging available
- ❑ **Has antibiotic prophylaxis been given within the last 60 minutes?**
  - Plan for redosing discussed

Briefing
- ❑ **Everyone please state your name and role.**

Surgeon discusses:
- ❑ Operative plan and possible difficulties
- ❑ Expected duration of procedure
- ❑ Anticipated blood loss
- ❑ Implants or special equipment needed

Anesthesia Provider discusses:
- ❑ Anesthetic plan
- ❑ Airway or other concerns

Nursing team discusses:
- ❑ Sterility, including indicator results
- ❑ Any equipment issues or other concerns

Surgeon states:
"Does anybody have any concerns? If you see something that concerns you during this case, please speak up."

Before Patient Leaves Room

Nurse reviews with team:
- ❑ Instrument, sponge and needle counts are correct
- ❑ Name of the procedure performed
- ❑ Specimen labeling
  - Read back specimen labeling including patient's name

Debriefing

Surgical Team Discusses:
- ❑ Equipment problems that need to be addressed.
- ❑ Key concerns for patient recovery and management
- ❑ If anything could have been done to make this case safer or more efficient

Fig. 1. South Carolina surgical safety checklist template. (*Adapted from* WHO Surgical Safety Checklist. Available at: http://www.who.int/patientsafety/safesurgery/en. © World Health Organization 2008. All rights reserved.)

BEFORE INDUCTION OF ANESTHESIA
Sign In
Anesthesia Safety Check Completed
Anesthesiologist Reviews (CRNAs may perform on IV Anesthesia cases)
Patient is confirmed as to:
 Identity
 Procedure
 Site
 Surgeon
 Consent (Obtained & Signed)
 Site Marked (if applicable)

Risk of hypothermia (operation >1 hour). If yes, warmer in place.

Does patient have *Allergies?*

Does patient take *beta blockers?*

Is surgeon available to begin once Anesthesia has been induced?

Has airway been assessed and special equipment available for anticipated airway issues?

Nursing Team Reviews
 SCD's in place
 Sterility Confirmed
 Is essential imaging displayed?
 Implants available?
 Other patient concerns

BEFORE SKIN INCISION
Time Out
Everyone stop what they are doing…
Surgeon Reviews
Team members introduce themselves by name and role
To follow cases with same staff – no introductions necessary. Whenever a change in staff occurs, introductions must be repeated.
Surgeon verbally confirms with the surgical team:
 • Patient
 • Site
 • Procedure
 • Position
 • Risk of > 500 ml blood loss (7ml/kg in children) If yes, adequate intravenous access and fluids planned
 • Does patient have allergies?

Anticipated Critical Events
Surgeon Reviews
Brief overall description of procedure and any anticipated difficulties
- Expected duration of procedure
- Single operative field vs. multiple operative fields
- Need for instruments/supplies beyond those normally used for the procedure.
Surgeon confirms with Anesthesia Team
Have antibiotics been given in the last 60 minutes?
Antibiotic redosing plan in place (not applicable <3 hrs)?
Beta Blocker given?
Glucose checked for Diabetics?
Surgeon confirms with Nursing Team
-Sterility Confirmed?
- Is essential imaging displayed?
- Implants available?
- Other patient concerns?

BEFORE SURGEON LEAVES OR
Sign Out
Surgeon verbally confirms with the team.
- Did we do all the procedures on the consent?
- The name of the procedure recorded
- That instrument, sponge and needle counts are correct (or not applicable)
- How the specimen is labeled (including patient name)
- Whether there are any equipment/problems to be addressed
- Neutral zone used? Any exposures?

All members of the surgical team review the key concerns for recovery and management of this patient.

Fig. 2. Surgical safety checklist used in the Greenville hospital system.

us a team that functions and communicates at an efficient level. I have seen how much teamwork can make a difference."

The South Carolina Checklist Template is shown in **Fig. 1**. This template was given to all of the hospitals involved in the introduction of checklists and was modified as needed.

The checklist used in the Greenville Hospital System is shown in **Fig. 2**. In contrast with the WHO checklist, checklists in the United States include items recommended in the Surgical Care

A   **UPON ENTERING THE OPERATING ROOM**
(RN, ST, CRNA)

✓ **Confirm patient identification**
-Name and date of birth

✓ **Do the procedure and consent agree?**

✓ **Are the posted equipment needs and outside providers available?**

✓ **Confirm the surgical site**
-What does the consent say?
-Does the patient agree?
-Is the site marked?

✓ **Does the patient have any known allergies?**

✓ **Does the patient have any contact or blood precautions?**

✓ **Is a difficult airway anticipated?**
-Are there alternative plans?
-Is the appropriate equipment available?
-Is there an increased risk for aspiration?

✓ **Are antibiotics on hand and begun?**

✓ **Was a beta blocker given?**

✓ **Is DVT prophylaxis indicated?**

✓ **Is the room warm enough?**

✓ **Anesthesia safety check**
-Machine
-Circuit
-Drugs
-Devices

B   **PRE-OP BRIEFING AND TIME OUT**
(ENTIRE TEAM)

✓ **Do we all know each other?**
-Each person introduce yourself at the beginning of day and with relief
-Record names on white board

✓ **Surgeon confirms:**
-Patient name
-Procedure
-Site
-Position
-Imaging
-Operative plan and potential difficulties
-Expected duration of procedure
-OP vs. admission
-Implants or special equipment
-Fire safety risk
   Alcohol containing preps dried (ChloraPrep)
   Head/neck procedures
   Open source of oxygen
-Anticipated blood loss
   If over 10%, anesthesia discusses IV access
   Is blood available and on hand
   Beginning Hgb/Hct

✓ **Anesthesia providers review:**
-Allergies
-Antibiotics
-Beta blocker
-DVT prophylaxis
-Temperature regulation
-Any post-op concerns
   Airway issues
   Analgesia
   ICU/specialty bed
   Isolation, blood precautions
"Does anyone have any concerns?
If you see something that concerns you during
this case, please speak up."

C   **END OF CASE DEBRIEFING**
(ENTIRE TEAM)

✓ **Are the counts correct?**

✓ **What is the name of the procedure that was performed?**
-What is the post-op diagnosis?
-Is the post-op diagnosis the same as the pre-op diagnosis?
-Did the wound class change?

✓ **Read back specimen labels**

✓ **Surgical team discusses:**
-Any changes to plans for recovery?
-Are antibiotics to be continued?
-Should beta blockers be continued?
-Are there equipment issues to be addressed?

✓ **Could anything have been done to make this case safer or more efficient?**

Fig. 3. Palmetto Health surgical safety checklist. DVT, deep venous thrombosis; Hct, hematocrit; Hgb, hemoglobin. (*Adapted from* WHO Surgical Safety Checklist. Available at: http://www.who.int/patientsafety/safesurgery/en. © World Health Organization 2008. All rights reserved.)

Improvement Project (SCIP): antibiotics given within 60 minutes of skin incision, patient warmer in place for operations longer than 1 hour, deep venous thrombosis prophylaxis.

Fig. 3 shows the checklist presently used in the Palmetto Health System, composed of 2 hospitals in Columbia: Palmetto Health Richland and Palmetto Health Baptist. Palmetto Heath Richland is

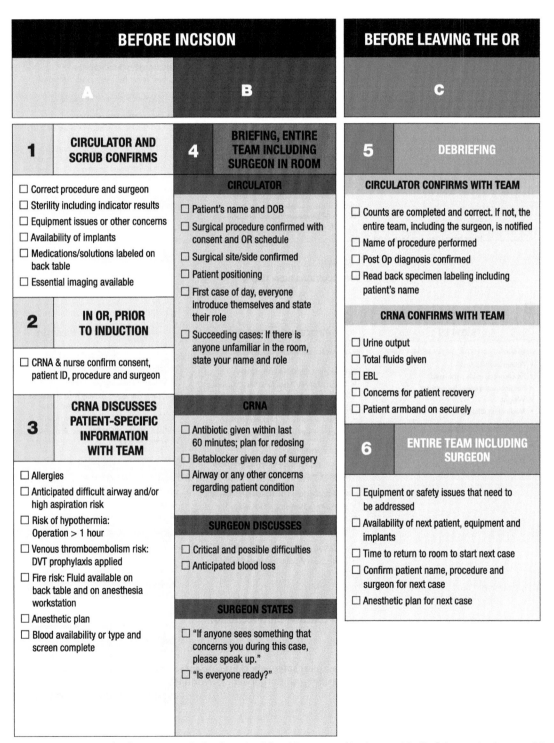

Fig. 4. Lexington Medical Center surgical safety checklist. (*Courtesy of* Lexington Medical Center, Lexington, SC; with permission.)

A

Before Induction of Anesthesia in OR	Before Skin Incision/Procedure	Before Patient Leaves OR
SIGN IN-INITIATED BY CIRCULATOR	**TIME OUT-INITIATED BY SURGEON**	**SIGN OUT-INITIATED BY SURGEON**

VERIFICATION STEPS VERBALIZED OUT LOUD FOR ALL TEAM MEMBERS TO REVIEW:

ANESTHESIOLOGIST & CIRCULATOR VERIFIES:
1. Patient Identification
   - Matching 2 identifiers with name band
   - Engage parents and patient (when applicable)
2. Procedure & Site/Side
   - Engage parents and patient (when applicable)
3. Site marked by surgeon performing procedure
4. Weight and Allergies

WHEN CLINICALLY INDICATED:
5. Compression boots used for DVT prophylaxis
6. Warmers in place to prevent hypothermia

ALL TEAM MEMBERS
1. Introduce self by name and role

SURGEON VERIFIES:
1. Patient/Procedure/Site/Side & Position
2. Critical Steps/Anticipated Risks/EBL/Duration
3. Special Equipment/Implants needed
4. Imaging, labs, and other relevant preoperative tests reviewed and available

ANESTHESIOLOGIST VERIFIES:
1. Antibiotics given within 60 min of incision
2. IV access appropriate for anticipated EBL
3. Blood (or cross-match) available if needed

CIRCULATING/SCRUB NURSE VERIFIES:
1. Consent matches verbalized procedure
2. Site marking visible in prepped field
3. Special Equipment/Implants available
4. Medications/Solutions labeled on field

STOP!
ANY QUESTIONS FROM TEAM?

SURGEON VERIFIES:
1. Name of procedure to be recorded

CIRCULATOR/SCRUB VERIFIES:
1. Final counts (sponge/instrument/needles)
2. Correct labeling of specimens
3. Equipment problems to be addressed

ALL TEAM MEMBERS DISCUSS:
1. Key concerns for postoperative period
2. Airway concerns during recovery
3. EBL and likelihood of ongoing blood loss
4. Need and timing for post-op labs/imaging
5. Plan for communicating key recovery issues to accepting team (safe hand-off)

B

SIGN IN	PROCEDURAL TIME OUT	WOUND CLOSURE TIME OUT

ANESTHESIOLOGIST & CIRCULATOR VERIFY:
- Patient identification
- Procedure(s) to be performed
- Surgical site marked by surgeon
- Weight
- Medication allergies

WHEN CLINICALLY INDICATED:
- DVT prophylaxis / Compression boots
- Warming devices in place

TEAM MEMBERS INTRODUCE NAME & ROLE

SURGEON & CIRCULATOR VERIFY:
- Correct Patient/Procedure/Site/Positioning
- Consent matches procedure(s)
- Site marking visible in surgical field
- Special equipment / Implants available
- Equipment settings (e.g. cautery/insufflation)

SURGEON VERIFIES:
- Critical steps of case reviewed with team
- Relevant imaging and labs reviewed

ANESTHESIOLOGIST & SURGEON VERIFIES:
- Antibiotic indication / Given within 1hr
- Re-dosing plan if duration >4hrs
- Blood (or cross-match) available if needed

CIRCULATOR & SCRUB PERSONNEL VERIFY:
- Medications / Solutions labeled on field

STOP!
ANY CONCERNS WITH PROCEEDING?

STOP!
CLOSING TIME OUT ANNOUNCED
- Wound exploration performed
- Counts completed audibly by both members of nursing team viewing counted items
- Team acknowledges closing count status
- Team initiates SIGN-OUT during or following wound closure

SIGN OUT

SURGEON VERIFIES:
- Name of procedure to be recorded
- Equipment problems to be addressed

ANESTHESIOLOGIST & SURGEON VERIFIES:
- Airway concerns during recovery
- EBL and likelihood of ongoing blood loss
- Fluids / Blood products administered
- Need and timing of post-op labs / Imaging
- Disposition and hand-off plans

CIRCULATOR VERIFIES:
- Final count (sponges/instruments/needles)
- Disposition/Correct labeling of all specimens

Fig. 5. Children's Hospital Boston pediatric surgical safety checklist. (*Adapted from* WHO Surgical Safety Checklist. Available at: http://www.who.int/patientsafety/safesurgery/en. © World Health Organization 2008. All rights reserved.)

C

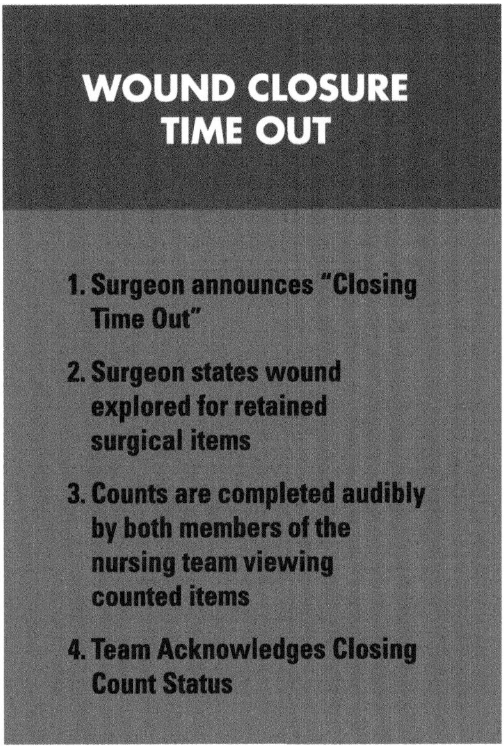

WOUND CLOSURE TIME OUT

1. Surgeon announces "Closing Time Out"

2. Surgeon states wound explored for retained surgical items

3. Counts are completed audibly by both members of the nursing team viewing counted items

4. Team Acknowledges Closing Count Status

Fig. 5. (*continued*)

the teaching hospital of the University of South Carolina School of Medicine. Composed of 3 pages, most of the checklist items on the first page are reviewed in the preoperative holding area before the patient enters the operating room.

Fig. 4 shows the checklist presently used at Lexington Medical Center (LMC) in Columbia, South Carolina, and includes the SCIP recommendations. LMC is a 414-bed community hospital in West Columbia, South Carolina, with more than 600 affiliated physicians. It offers a complete range of surgical services, including cardiac and neurosurgery. The same checklist is used in all of the operating rooms.

Pediatric patients are usually not able to participate in identifying the site of surgery. As a result, Boston Children's Hospital developed a surgical checklist specific for the pediatric population, which is shown in **Fig. 5**. Norton and Rangl[22] reviewed the introduction of the checklist at Boston Children's Hospital and found that it improved teamwork, communication, and adherences to processes. Checklists were also developed in other areas of the hospital where invasive procedures were performed. This article also includes pediatric procedural and pediatric bedside safety checklists.

Another useful checklist is depicted on the Web site of the Association of Perioperative Registered Nurses (www.aorn.org). This checklist includes color-coded items that indicate their origin: WHO, Joint Commission, universal protocols, and both Joint Commission and WHO.

EXTENSION OF THE SURGICAL CHECKLIST TO OUTPATIENT SURGERY

The Center for Medicare and Medicaid Service (CMS) has indicated that, in 2013, ambulatory surgical centers (ASCs) will be required to go to the CMS Quality Net Web site between July 1 and August 15 and report whether they used a safe-surgery checklist at any time between January 1, 2012, and December 31, 2012, for all patients, not just those covered by Medicare.

ASCs are required to report safe surgery practices during each of the 3 critical perioperative periods. Because CMS is not dictating that ASCs use a particular checklist, ASCs are free to select a checklist (or multiple checklists) that meets their need. Although CMS uses the name safe surgery checklist, the measure applies to all ASC procedures, including those that are generally considered to be diagnostic and pain management procedures (eg, certain endoscopies and injections for controlling pain).[23,24]

I frequently operate at Parkridge Surgery Center (PSC), an ambulatory surgical center that was the first ASC in South Carolina to adopt the checklist. One of the physician champions is Chad Rubin, MD, a general surgeon in Columbia. I spoke to Dr Rubin about the changes between PSCs checklist and the other checklists in use in inpatient facilities. This checklist is shown in **Fig. 6**.

Newkirk: "How was the surgical checklist now used at Parkridge Surgery Center developed?"

Rubin: "Parkridge Surgery Center was the first ASC to adopt a checklist in South Carolina. We took the checklist that we thought was most applicable to outpatient surgery and modified it. It has the key items that are important for us to know. [We do a lot of plastic surgery and ophthalmology at the surgicenter] so we included a part on whether or not we needed implants and are they available. We dropped the portion related to administration of blood.

I think that's what's even more important is that everybody identifies themselves; they tell who they are and what their role is. This often occurs when you are gowning and gloving and takes very little time. The

Before Skin Incision

Surgeon, Nurse, and Anesthesia Provider perform the Time Out:
- ❑ Patient's name
- ❑ Patient Allergies
- ❑ Patient Positioning/pressure points checked

Verify from consent and H&P:
- ❑ Surgical procedure to be performed
- ❑ Surgical site
- ❑ **Has antibiotic prophylaxis been given within the last 60 minutes?**

Briefing

- ❑ **Everyone please state your name and role.**
  (first thing in the morning and with relief)

Surgeon discusses:
- ❑ Any changes to operative plan and possible difficulties

Anesthesia Provider discusses:
- ❑ Anesthetic plan
- ❑ Airway or other concerns

Nursing team discusses:
- ❑ Any equipment issues or other concerns
- ❑ All medications correct and labeled
- ❑ Confirms correct implants

Surgeon states:
"Does anybody have any concerns? If you see something that concerns you during this case, please speak up."

Before Patient Leaves Room

Nurse reviews with team:
- ❑ Instrument, sponge and needle counts are correct
- ❑ Name of the procedure performed
- ❑ Specimen labeling
  - ➡ Read back specimen labeling including patient's name

Debriefing

Surgical Team Discusses:
- ❑ Equipment problems that need to be addressed.
- ❑ Key concerns for patient recovery and management
- ❑ If anything could have been done to make this case safer or more efficient

Fig. 6. South Carolina surgical safety checklist template. (*Courtesy of* Palmetto Health, Columbia, SC; with permission.)

anesthetist introduces herself and you ask what are you using as an anesthetic? Do you think we are going to have problems?

Then you go to the circulating nurse, whose role is giving the time out, do we have the right patient? Are we doing the right procedure? Then you bring the techs in: do we have the right equipment? Do we have the right anesthetic on the field? You have everybody involved.

The most important question is you ask is, 'Does anyone have any concerns?' Ninety-nine point nine percent of the time nobody has any concerns, but it changes the atmosphere in the entire operating room, I am absolutely convinced it brings more of a team approach: [As a team member] I'm not afraid to speak up."

Newkirk: "Has the use of the checklist prevented any mishaps?"

Rubin: "I keep going back to this example, but it's an incredible example. We went through the checklist, and this was fairly early on at the outpatient surgery center. I was doing a left inguinal hernia repair. The patient had had previous surgery. The consent said that we are doing a recurrent left inguinal hernia repair, and the tech spoke up and said, 'But Dr Rubin, the scar is on the right.' I said, 'Whoa, let's stop, let's go back and go through the chart.' As it turns out, the patient had had bilateral inguinal hernia repairs and the recurrence was on the left but, amazingly, you couldn't see the scar on the left, but you could see it on the right. That's the kind of culture that you want to have: it was the tech that spoke up, who probably wouldn't have spoken up if we didn't have this kind of atmosphere."

SUMMARY

It is clear that the use of surgical checklists decreases complications and saves lives. After reviewing the literature I have concluded that that the use of a checklist causes a major positive improvement in surgical culture. This improvement will benefit patients and physicians. The American Association for Ambulatory Surgical Facilities, Inc, now mandates that a surgical checklist be used prior to surgical procedures using sedation or general anesthesia.

ACKNOWLEDGMENT

I would like to thank Lisa Antley-Hearn, MLIS, Coordinator of library services, Lexington Medical Center, for helping me research this article.

REFERENCES

1. Meilinger PS. When the fortress went down. Air Force Magazine 2004;78–82.
2. Wenzel RP, Edmond MB. Team-based prevention of catheter-related infections. N Engl J Med 2006;355: 2781–3.
3. Pronovost P, Needham D, Berenholtz S, et al. An intervention to decrease catheter-related bloodstream infections in the ICU. N Engl J Med 2006;355:2725–32.
4. National nosocomial infections surveillance system, data summary January 1992 through June 2004. Am J Infect Control 2004;32:470–85.
5. Gwande A. The checklist manifesto. New York: Metropolitan Books; 2009. p. 39.
6. Weiser TG, Regenbogen SE, Thompson BA, et al. An estimation of the global volume of surgery: a modeling strategy based on available data. Lancet 2008;372(9633):139–44.
7. Available at: http://www.who.int/patientsafety/events/07/safer_surgery_summary_notes.pdf.
8. Haynes AB, Weiser TG, Berry WR, et al. A surgical safety checklist to reduce morbidity and mortality in a global population. N Engl J Med 2009;360:491–9.
9. Weiser TG, Haynes AB, Lashower A, et al. Int J Qual Health Care 2010;1–6.
10. Martin IC, Mason M, Findlay G. N Engl J Med 2009; 360:2272–3.
11. McCambridge J, Kypri K, Elbourne DR. N Engl J Med 2009;360:2373.
12. Sanders RD, Jameson SS. N Engl J Med 2009;360: 2373.
13. Haynes AB, Gwande AA. N Engl J Med 2009;360: 2374–5.
14. van Klei WA, Hoff RG, van Aarnhem EE, et al. Effects of the introduction of the WHO "Surgical Safety Checklist" in in-hospital mortality. Ann Surg 2012; 255(1):44–9.
15. Neily J, Mills PD, Young-Xu Y, et al. Association between implementation of a medical team training program and surgical mortality. JAMA 2010; 304(15):1693–700.
16. De Vries EN, Prins HA, Rogier MP, et al. Effect of a comprehensive surgical safety system on patient outcomes. N Engl J Med 2010;363: 1928–37.
17. De Vries EN, Hollmann MW, Smorenburg SM, et al. Development and validation on the SURgical Patient Safety System (SURPASS) checklist. Qual Saf Health Care 2009;18:121–6.
18. Birkmeyer JD. Strategies for improving surgical quality-checklists and beyond. N Engl J Med 2010; 363:1963–5.
19. De Vries EN, Dijkstra L, Smorenburg SM, et al. Patient Saf Surg 2010;4:106.
20. Available at: www.safesurgery2015.org.
21. William Berry, MD, speech at SCHA, October 17, 2012.
22. Norton EK, Rangl SJ. Implementing a pediatric surgical safety checklist in the OR and beyond. AORN J 2010;92:61–71.
23. ASCA News, 11/22/2011. Available at: www.ascassociation.org.
24. Available at: http://oregonpatientsafety.org. Accessed September 17, 2012.

Mandate for Accreditation in Plastic Surgery Ambulatory/ Outpatient Clinics

Jeff Pearcy, MPA, CAE*, Thomas Terranova, MA

KEYWORDS

- History of accreditation • Plastic surgery ambulatory clinics • JCAH • AAAHC • AAAASF
- Medicare

KEY POINTS

- Efforts at patient safety are integrated with Medicare requirements.
- Plastic surgeons have taken a lead in patient safety.
- The future of patient safety will depend on data-driven analysis.

BACKGROUND

Patient safety in ambulatory surgery settings has evolved through a combination of state/federal regulation, private accreditation, and increased patient awareness.

A function of state government is the protection of the public. The control of the practice of medicine is a primary exercise of this function. This control is exhibited both in the licensing of those who may practice medicine and in the settings in which it can be practiced. Legal precedent for the privatization of public protection functions exists in a variety of decisions by both state and federal courts.

Technological advances have allowed health care services to migrate across settings increasingly outside of the hospital, and regulatory jurisdictions have the unenviable obligation to protect a public receiving care in more numerous and diverse facilities. From the regulatory perspective, ambulatory surgery encompasses outpatient health care facilities ranging from large multi-suite ambulatory surgery centers to single-physician procedure rooms. Although cosmetic and plastic surgery receive a disproportionate amount of media and legislator attention, concerns related to outpatient care and oversight are not unique to any specialty. Government agencies have the ultimate responsibility to ensure the safety of their constituents and have increasingly turned to private accrediting bodies to establish a comprehensive regulatory program partnering state enforcement authority and private survey capabilities. Twenty-seven states now accept or mandate accreditation in at least one of the ambulatory settings.

PRIVATE ACCREDITATION EVOLUTION

Historically, "Professional societies began regulating medical practice by examining and licensing practitioners as early as 1760. By the early 1800s, the medical societies were in charge of establishing regulations, standards of practice, and certification of doctors."[1] As medical education and regulation began to mature, care began to migrate from the home to the hospital. Emanuel Codman, MD, first proposed for the standardization of hospitals in 1910. The first set of requirements was developed by the American College of Surgeons

Author Disclosures: Both authors are employees of the American Association for Accreditation of Ambulatory Surgery Facilities, Inc.

The American Association for Accreditation of Ambulatory Surgery Facilities, Inc, 5101 Washington Street, Gurnee, IL 60031, USA

* Corresponding author.

E-mail address: jeff@aaaasf.org

Clin Plastic Surg 40 (2013) 489–492

http://dx.doi.org/10.1016/j.cps.2013.04.012

in 1917: a 1-page document.[2] Accreditation mandates in ambulatory surgery are legacies inherited from hospital oversight. The manner in which regulatory oversight is delegated by government to third-party agencies approximates hospital oversight regimen that began with the Hospital Standardization Program in the early part of the twentieth century and formalized with mandated Joint Commission accreditation for Medicare-participating hospitals in 1965. Delegation of authority has followed the decentralization of health care services because it is quite effective for government to identify private regulatory partners whereby public agencies may have a particular weakness or limitation. "The American College of Physicians, the American Hospital Association, the American Medical Association and the Canadian Medical Association joined with the American College of Surgeons as corporate members to create the joint commission on accreditation of Hospitals in 1951."[2] In 1965 The Joint Commission on Accreditation of Healthcare Organizations (JCAHO) was recognized in the Social Security Amendments to provide accreditation of hospitals.

Federal regulatory efforts lagged behind the changes in the provisions of health care. In the early 1970s there was a significant migration of health care and surgical services from the hospital to neighborhood regional ambulatory centers. JCAH at the time did not provide a program of accreditation for these centers. To meet this need, the Accreditation for Ambulatory Health Care was incorporated in Illinois.[3]

In 1980 the American Society of Plastic and Reconstructive Surgeons recognized that surgeons operating in freestanding facilities were unable to access accreditation through JCAH or Accreditation for Ambulatory Health Care and established the American Association for Ambulatory Plastic Surgery Facilities to design and operate a single-specialty accreditation program for outpatient plastic surgery centers. Based on inquiries by other surgical specialties, the American Association for Ambulatory Plastic Surgery Facilities formed the American Association for Accreditation of Ambulatory Surgery Facilities (AAAASF) in 1992 to accredit other single-specialty and multispecialty surgery facilities, owned and operated by physicians certified by the American Board of Medical Specialties. AAAASF currently accredits facilities that include all the American Board of Medical Specialties surgical disciplines.

This evolution is consistent with other business sectors requiring specialized knowledge, because agencies often rely on regulation by private arm's length organizations with expertise in the subject matter. Health care facilities, prisons, and institutions of higher learning are commonly associated with private accreditation, not surprising given that the concepts related to administering such institutions are likely to be foreign to most people outside of those fields. Accreditation organizations are representative of the industries they regulate; thus, the people setting and revising standards work in the field and are at the forefront of research, driving the latest developments in quality and safety.

Deferring to private accreditation is, at least in part, an acknowledgment of the institutional inertia that can delay regulatory changes. Although it is certainly possible for a public agency to create its own set of standards, it is less probable for that agency to keep up with the rapid developments of the industry. Revision attempts slow considerably due to political negotiations, bureaucratic review processes, and public comment periods. Competing interests each have the opportunity to voice their opinions during the public revision process, sometimes yielding few rewards. The original Medicare hospital conditions for participation were published in 1966; attempted updates to the conditions began in 1977 but were not finalized until 1986. The Centers for Medicare and Medicaid Services published its first major revisions to the ambulatory surgery center conditions for coverage in mid-2008, 26 years after the initial adoption. By contrast, accreditation organizations typically revisit their standards annually to at least study minor adjustments, if not to undertake wholesale revisions.

Federal and state agencies' biggest impetus for delegating to accreditation agencies may be cost. Administering an inspection and certification regime is a costly enterprise in financial and personnel terms. Private organizations can often realize cost efficiencies that are impossible for government agencies and can therefore perform inspections with lower operating costs. Many states have statutory limits or prohibitions on fees that a facility may be charged. Higher costs and budgetary limits exert extraordinary pressure on government programs. In 1991 Medicare estimated that internally administering the hospital certification program would require 722 additional full-time personnel, an increase of nearly one-third, and $59 million in operating costs that would have to be absorbed into the budget.[4] The state of Washington administers a portion of its Ambulatory Surgery Facility licensing and inspection program, performing at least 1 of the 2 surveys that each facility must complete in each 36-month period. The state department of health identified that its initial cost and personnel estimates for operating the licensing program were shorter than the actual needs and was able to secure statutory authority to raise licensing fees and add staff. The result is a new tiered licensing fee structure with a maximum 3-year fee of $10,068, or $5410 if the facility is accredited. Private accreditation agencies charge fees directly to facilities; thus, they are not in such a precarious financial position and are able to adjust staff accordingly.

Simple efficiency certainly plays a role in government's willingness to accept or mandate accreditation in lieu of a state process. In the mid-1990s the 2 major US plastic surgery societies (American Society for Aesthetic Plastic Surgery and the American Society of Plastic Surgeons and The American Society of Plastic and Reconstructive Surgeons) mandated that all members operate only in licensed or accredited facilities. This mandate was a critical turning point for plastic surgery as well as for accreditation. The mandate was a demonstration to medical boards and public advocates of the specialty's commitment to quality and safety. Continuing to operate in the office, terrifyingly called unlicensed facilities, as many plastic surgeons did, only put their reputations and professional licenses at risk. As more jurisdictions considered regulating all outpatient settings, the existing foundation of specialty mandated accreditation must have presented an attractive option for regulatory oversight without adding a redundant inspection process.

LEGISLATIVE EVOLUTION

California led the way in officially mandating accreditation. In 1995 the California legislature passed Assembly Bill 595, requiring oversight over all outpatient settings using anesthesia at higher levels than local anesthesia. The primary mechanism for office surgery, those facilities not licensed through the state and not participating in Medicare, to achieve requisite oversight became accreditation. Contemporary articles explain the state's patient safety concerns and the legislature emphasized that the intent of Bill 595 was to "assure that the least costly and effective method of achieving patient safety is required." The bill was initially drafted in response to increased commercial advertisement for office-based cosmetic surgery but gained traction after the death of a pediatric patient under anesthesia. California had a duty to ensure that those physicians advertising for cosmetic surgery were properly trained and qualified to provide those services; without the personnel and financial resources to survey every one of the offices in question, the state favored mandatory accreditation. Passing the law became a moral imperative with the young patient's unfortunate passing.

When one considers the impetus for regulation as noted above with the administrative challenges extant for most state and federal agencies, detailed in the previous section, it is only logical that states would prefer a delegated form of regulatory oversight. In this model the government can devote its valuable resources to investigating complaints or adverse incidents and assuring the quality of accrediting organizations that it approves to perform the oversight function. Thus the state only has to perform a handful of routine reviews of accrediting organizations rather than surveying hundreds or potentially thousands of facilities. The result is a more efficient use of public resources and an effective method to assure quality and safety.

Scenarios similar to California's have occurred across the country with largely the same results. A tragic event or the aggregation of several lower impact events cause increased media coverage and foment legislative resolve to protect the public. Traditionally the resulting regulatory regimes subject facilities to oversight with sedation or higher levels of anesthesia use. Adverse events pertaining to plastic surgery are particularly attractive as media stories and receive tremendous public attention because the patients affected are typically healthy when they elect to undergo a procedure. Any resulting long-term damage is particularly compelling. Complications are only exacerbated if the operating physician performs a procedure outside of their specialty training. An attractive feature of accreditation is that every approved accreditation agency has methods by which physicians prove appropriate training and competency in the specialties performed in the facility.

Despite the high-profile nature of complications related to plastic surgery and specialty drift, there are myriad patient safety issues related to the routine provision of care in every medical specialty. The 2008 hepatitis exposure of patients in 2 Nevada gastroenterology facilities is a prime example. The cases were related to improper injection practices and insufficient infection control oversight, not physicians operating outside of their scopes of practice. The resulting regulatory regime requires both state inspection and accreditation of all outpatient facilities.

The emerging trend in mandatory accreditation is to combine oversight based on the level of anesthesia used with enumerating procedures that require accreditation. Unfortunately some physicians have attempted to skirt regulatory requirements by providing inappropriate care under local anesthesia, which not only complicates matters for physicians providing appropriate care in the form of procedures that can be safely performed under local anesthesia but it also frustrates the efforts of regulators who want to ensure patient safety without overburdening physicians that are safely performing minor procedures under local anesthetic in the office. Proposed solutions include adding mandated accreditation for certain listed procedures most commonly associated with untoward events, no matter what level of anesthetic is used, to existing anesthesia-based requirements. Regulators hope the hybrid approach will discourage unscrupulous practitioners from bypassing rules by dangerously operating under local anesthesia, without overburdening those safely operating within their specialty.

FUTURE REGULATORY TRENDS IN ACCREDITATION

As early as 1994 Timothy Stotzfus Jost predicted a new role for the private accrediting bodies. "If the Joint Commission can establish itself as a credible source measuring quality, it may in the future find that its primary customers are not the institutions it accredits, the doctors who work in those institutions, or the government, but rather the consumers of health care and their institutional agents or the an agent and adviser of purchasers."[5]

A revolution in information has occurred for patients seeking to have more access to a wide variety of information regarding their health. They are bombarded by information in the form of commercials identifying diseases and treatments that they are encouraged to discuss with their physicians. The Internet search engines provide a library of information on every imaginable disease and surgical intervention. This information is seldom based on scientific fact, but becomes a part of fact by frequency.

At the same time that there is this increase in information, there has been a shortage of actual data that measure outcomes controlled for specific interventions. AAAASF has pioneered this type of data collection and analysis by instituting mandated reporting of adverse incidents in all surgical cases. The future of patient safety and accreditation will depend on the evolution of the ability to mine patient safety data from electronic medical records and surgical notes.

The trend seems to couple outcomes data with performance-based purchasing of health care. This next shift in regulation and accreditation may provide adequate information to the consumer and the payer of health care to make decisions based on location of services, patient safety, quality of the care experience, and cost.

REFERENCES

1. Medline, Institute of Medicine. Available at: http://www.nlm.nih.gov/medlineplus/ency/article/001936.htm. Accessed April 12, 2013.
2. The Joint Commission. Available at: http://www.jointcommission.org/assets/1/6/Joint_Commission_History_2012.pdf. Accessed April 12, 2013.
3. Accreditation Association for Ambulatory Health Care, Inc. Available at: https://www.aaahc.org/Global/pdfs/Content%20from%202012%20Handbooks/D_History%20of%20AAAHC.pdf. Accessed April 12, 2013.
4. Havighurst CC. Private accreditation in the regulatory state. Duke University School of Law. Law Contemp Probl 1994;57(4):1–14.
5. Jost TS. Medicare and the Joint Commission on Accreditation of Healthcare Organizations: a healthy relationship?. Duke University School of Law. Law Contemp Probl 1994;57(4):15–45.

International Accreditation of Ambulatory Surgical Centers and Medical Tourism

Michael F. McGuire, MD[a,b,*]

KEYWORDS

- Accreditation • Ambulatory surgical centers • Outpatient surgery • International accreditation
- Plastic surgery • Outpatient facilities • Medical tourism • Patient safety

KEY POINTS

- The two forces that have driven the increase in accreditation of outpatient ambulatory surgery centers (ASC's) in the United States are reimbursement of facility fees by Medicare and commercial insurance companies, which requires either accreditation, Medicare certification, or state licensure, and state laws which mandate one of these three options.
- Accreditation of ASC's internationally has been driven by national requirements and by the competitive forces of "medical tourism." The three American accrediting organizations have all developed international programs to meet this increasing demand outside of the United States.

INTRODUCTION

Over the past decade, there has been an increasing interest on the part of many aspects of American medicine to become more involved with international colleagues, from the interest of the Accreditation Council on Graduate Medical Education and the American Board of Medical Specialties in exploring opportunities in international residency training and board certification to the development by many medical specialty organizations of increased relationships with international counterparts. Simultaneously, the growth of medical tourism has been driven by commercial insurance payers and corporations as well as by individuals to obtain medical care abroad at cheaper rates or to obtain procedures or drugs not yet available in the United States. This situation has also spurred domestic interest in foreign medicine and surgery.

There is a long history of the international involvement of American physicians in medical missions, medical education, international medical organizations, fellowship study abroad, and rich collegial interactions, but more recently there has been a realization that there is increased quality and sophistication in medicine around the world, as well as a growing desire both in the United States and in many other countries to increase professional interaction for mutually beneficial goals. These newer initiatives have been based on recognition of the similarity of challenges confronting physicians in all parts of the world, and the value of sharing experiences and solutions. In some areas, the United States has had successes in solving problems, or has developed programs that may be of value to our international colleagues; in many other areas, various other countries have had greater successes in dealing with challenges or developed a more innovative

[a] Department of Surgery, Division of Plastic Surgery, University of Southern California, 1520 San Pablo Street, Los Angeles, CA 90033 USA; [b] Department of Surgery, Division of Plastic Surgery, University of California, Los Angeles, 757 Westwood Plaza, Los Angeles, CA 90095, USA
* 1301 20th Street, Suite 460, Santa Monica, CA 90404, USA.
E-mail address: mmcguire@UCLA.edu

Clin Plastic Surg 40 (2013) 493–498
http://dx.doi.org/10.1016/j.cps.2013.04.013
0094-1298/13/$ – see front matter © 2013 Published by Elsevier Inc.

approach that we can benefit from in the United States. Unlike many older relationships, in which the United States tended to dominate and control the activities and focus of an international exchange, the more recent approach has been more collegial, more equal, and more focused on mutual benefit.

THE INCREASE OF MANDATORY ACCREDITATION OF AMBULATORY SURGICAL CENTERS

In the United States, the accreditation of outpatient surgical facilities, especially those not part of an acute care hospital, has slowly become important, and, in many cases, mandatory, for several reasons.

Federal Medicare Program

The federal Medicare program began to certify out-of-hospital ambulatory surgical centers (ASCs) and reimburse them for facility fees in 1982 after developing and publishing the conditions for coverage (CfCs) in the Federal Register. These requirements form the fundamentals for determining which facilities can participate as a supplier under the Medicare program.[1] These CfCs have undergone numerous revisions and refinements over the ensuing years.

Three National Accrediting Organizations

Beginning in 1996, the Centers for Medicare and Medicaid Services (CMS, then called the Healthcare Financing Authority) began to allow the 3 national accrediting organizations to deem compliance with the CfCs for ASCs by an approved inspection process. This system was separate from the state agency process, which had been the only option to achieve Medicare certification before that time.[2]

The 3 organizations (the American Association for the Accreditation of Ambulatory Surgery Facilities [AAAASF], the Joint Commission, and the Accreditation Association for Ambulatory Health Care [AAAHC]) had to be approved by CMS as a deeming agency by showing that their standards and processes met or exceeded the CfCs for ASCs. That approval must be renewed by CMS every 6 years.

Outcomes of Compliance Process

This new process of deeming compliance dramatically improved the inspection system for ASCs seeking to participate in the Medicare program and made the requirements more uniform across all the states. The lengthy and variable delays in arranging site inspections under the state programs were virtually eliminated, and the number of certified facilities steadily increased. In 2011, the last year of available data, there were 5368 Medicare-certified ASCs, with continued growth over the last 3 years despite the economic slowdown.

The ASC payment system underwent a substantial revision in 2008, most significantly increasing the number of surgical procedures that would be covered.

More than 3500 surgical procedures are covered by the Medicare system in certified ASCs. However, payments from Medicare are not a substantial source of revenue for most ASCs. A study by the Medical Group Management Association in 2009, for example, showed that only 17% of ASC revenue was from Medicare, on average.[3] Commercial insurance reimbursement was the greatest source of revenue, but in many states Medicare certification is required to collect facility fees from commercial insurers.

Effect of State Laws on Accredited Surgical Facilities

The other factor that has increased the number of accredited surgical facilities has been the gradual increase in state laws requiring that all outpatient surgical centers be accredited by 1 of the 3 national organizations, certified by Medicare, or licensed by the state. This movement began in California in 1995, when the state began to evaluate the need for some oversight of the burgeoning ambulatory surgery industry, which had no requirements for operating until that time.

Unlike the situation in acute care hospitals, which have long had extensive requirements covering all aspects of patient care, including safety, sterility, personnel, physical plant, and so forth, the outpatient center could start caring for patients, administering general anesthesia, and performing major surgery without anyone inspecting the facility or certifying compliance with even basic requirements.

The new law went into effect in July, 1996 in California,[4] and has been followed by laws in 21 states that mandate either state licensure, accreditation by 1 of the 3 national organizations, or certification by Medicare. However, this situation means that there are still no requirements for these outpatient surgical centers in 28 states: no oversight, no inspection process, no standards to comply with, no control over what is performed in these facilities. In several states, laws have been proposed, and rejected by the regulatory agencies as unnecessary because there have been no reported deaths or serious complications as yet from these centers. Although elective surgery on generally healthy patients is inherently safe, as the types of procedures that are performed on an outpatient basis increase, and the health requirements for patients who qualify for surgery in ASCs decrease, it is inevitable that untoward outcomes will occur without some basic standards in place. Numerous studies have shown the safety of even major surgery performed in accredited facilities,[5–8] but without external oversight, the risks can increase to a dangerous level. The reluctance to act until a crisis occurs has meant that most states still have no protections in place to assure their citizens that basic requirements have been met when they have surgery and anesthesia in an outpatient surgical center.

The 2 major forces that have driven the requirement for accreditation of outpatient ambulatory surgery centers in the United States are:

1. Reimbursement of facility fees by Medicare and commercial insurance companies, which requires either accreditation, Medicare certification, or state licensure
2. State laws that mandate 1 of those 3 options for all centers

Impact of Professional Plastic Surgery Societies on Accredited Surgical Facilities

An additional strong incentive for plastic surgeons to operate only in accredited, Medicare-certified, or state-licensed facilities is the requirement for membership in the 2 largest national plastic surgery societies, the American Society of Plastic Surgeons, and the American Society for Aesthetic Plastic Surgery, that all outpatient surgery other than those performed under just local anesthesia is performed only in such facilities.[9,10] The American Board of Plastic Surgery (ABPS) now also requires compliance with this requirement as a part of the Maintenance of Certification program, which is mandatory for all diplomates certified after 1995. As a result, virtually all plastic surgeons certified by the ABPS operate only in these inspected surgery centers, whether or not their state requires it, and whether or not Medicare or commercial insurance cover the procedures that they are performing. This situation adds a measure of reassurance to patients considering elective surgery procedures, especially aesthetic surgery, in that they now know that not only is the surgeon performing the procedure appropriately trained and ABPS Board certified to perform it safely but the facility where it is being done is also certified as meeting national standards for patient safety and quality care.

International Facility Accreditation

None of these forces acting to require some degree of external oversight of the functions of an ASC exists internationally. Although some nations have imposed mandatory compliance with national standards, including France, the United Kingdom, Brazil, Australia, and Germany, most nations have no requirements in place. A recent effort to develop an ASC accreditation requirement in the European Union (based largely on the AAAASF model) has yet to materialize, caught up in the political turmoil that limits that group's efforts in so many areas. With so many more serious issues to confront in most nations, regulating ambulatory surgery centers is not even being considered. The Swiss Society of Plastic, Reconstructive, and Aesthetic Surgery recently mandated that surgery performed by its members outside of licensed hospitals must be done in ambulatory surgical facilities that have been inspected and accredited by the international affiliate of AAAASF, known as AAAASF-I.

THE MOVEMENT TOWARD AN OUTREACH ABROAD TO ACCREDIT SURGERY CENTERS

Recognizing the lack of any established programs to accredit hospitals and surgery centers internationally, the Joint Commission made the first venture into international accreditation in 1994, when it formed the Joint Commission International (JCI). Their program includes separate standards for multiple types of international health care organizations: ambulatory care, clinical laboratory, home care, hospital, long-term care, medical transport, primary care centers, and the Certification for Clinical Care Program (CCPC) which is focused on recognizing excellence in the integration and coordination of care for the treatment of specific diseases. There is no accreditation specifically for ambulatory surgery centers. Instead, all ambulatory care centers are grouped together, and the ambulatory care standards are applicable to a wide variety of organizations, including freestanding medical, surgical, and dental facilities, dialysis facilities, diagnostic radiology centers, chronic care management facilities. As a result, the standards are generic, with little detail regarding requirements for performing surgery or dental surgery in an ambulatory setting.

The JCI has now accredited or certified more than 400 organizations in 50 countries. However, most of these facilities are in the hospital category, and many of the accredited ambulatory facilities are nonsurgical. The number of accredited hospitals and other facilities in various countries can be directly related to the country's prominence in seeking to attract international patients for medical and surgical treatments, as is the number of CCPC certificates in those specialties with a special attraction for international patients. Countries such as India, Korea, Singapore, Thailand, Indonesia, and the United Arab Emirates have many JCI-accredited facilities and certified specialties. In some cases, the national governments are involved in encouraging hospitals and other facilities to obtain JCI accreditation as a part of their initiatives to encourage foreign medical tourists for economic benefits.[11]

In 2005, AAAASF recognized the potential of an international accreditation program for ambulatory surgical facilities. At the time, it was perceived that an organization with American in its name might not be welcomed in many nations, for political and economic reasons. Because there was also a need to keep the international program legally separate from the domestic activity of AAAASF, a subsidiary organization was formed similar to JCI. Surgery Facilities Resources was incorporated in 2005. The existing domestic standards for accreditation were modified to accommodate international cultural and social differences and maintain the high bar set by AAAASF, which has given it a reputation as the gold standard in accreditation. In 2009, as the program gained international recognition, and the value of accreditation by an American organization to facilities interested in attracting American patients for dental or surgical care became important, the name of the organization was changed to AAAASF International (AAAASF-I). The number of accredited dental and surgical facilities has grown steadily over the past 5 years, especially in Central and South America, as a result of intense competition to attract foreign patients as well as encouragement or requirement for accreditation by some national governments. There are now more than 115 ambulatory surgery and dental facilities accredited by AAAASF-I in 12 countries around the world, including the United States; the value of an international accreditation is recognized for marketing purposes, both domestically and internationally. The program has been endorsed by the International Society for Aesthetic Plastic Surgery and has trained inspectors to perform accrediting surveys in many countries.

More recently, AAAHC has formed an international subsidiary, and has just started to accredit facilities in Costa Rica and Peru. This increase in international accreditation has been motivated by several factors: the desire on the part of individual facilities as well as governments to attract foreign patients and the increasing demand for quality and safety in ambulatory surgery, both by international patients as well as by international governments, similar to the situation in the United States.

MEDICAL TOURISM

The concept of traveling abroad to obtain medical or surgical care, commonly termed medical tourism, dates back to the ancient Greeks, who traveled to seek the help of the god of medicine, Asclepius. Historically, medical travel was most often associated with wealthy citizens of less-developed countries going to more developed nations, because of the greater safety and quality of care in those nations. The United States and the United Kingdom were the destination of much of this medical travel, and Brazil has also long attracted patients desiring aesthetic plastic surgery, because of the quality of the surgeons. More recently, the travel patterns have been reversed, with many patients leaving the United States and the United Kingdom to receive surgery in many less-developed countries around the world.

Newer devices or drugs may not be available in the United States because of the lengthy approval process of the US Food and Drug Administration. Commercial insurers or Medicare may not cover newer techniques, such as stem cell therapies, because they are considered experimental, and they are often available abroad sooner.

Cost Factor

Cost, rather than quality, has been the principal motivation for this more recent travel. Also, in some cases, surgical procedures still considered experimental in the United States (and therefore not yet covered by commercial health insurers or Medicare) are only available abroad. In countries such as Canada and the United Kingdom, with national health systems, the long waiting lists that exist for less urgent surgery have also been a major motivation for seeking care abroad.

Although aesthetic surgery has been a significant part of the medical travel industry, increasingly, medically necessary surgery has been the more important component. Interest in procedures such as coronary bypass, hip and knee replacement, and organ transplant surgery covered by Medicare and third-party insurers has come from those in the United States who lose their employer-sponsored coverage from job loss or insurance coverage discontinuation by their employer. The millions of Americans without insurance coverage seek care internationally because the cost of these major surgeries abroad is estimated to be one-tenth or less of the cost in the United States, including round-trip air fare and postoperative recovery in a hotel or resort.[12]

Commercial Insurer-Driven Procedures Abroad

Some commercial insurers have developed programs to encourage their subscribers to go abroad to have their covered procedures performed, because of the cost savings to the company. Often, the insurers waive copayments and deductibles if surgery is performed abroad, and sometimes they even pay for travel expenses and companion travel. Blue Shield of California started Access Baja in 2000, directing patients to several hospitals in Mexico, and in 2007, Blue Cross/Blue Shield of South Carolina teamed up with hospitals in multiple foreign countries to provide care for subscribers. Some large employers who are self-insured have also developed programs to encourage their employees to seek surgery abroad, and this has been a major element in the development of the medical tourism industry.

Several individuals with a background in employee benefits management started one of the leading organizations promoting medical tourism, and a major focus of their meetings is to connect medical tourism facilitators with commercial insurers and employee benefits managers.

These medical tourism facilitators or concierges come from a variety of backgrounds. Many are travel agents, some are physicians or nurses, and others have experience in the insurance industry. They assist patients in finding providers of the medical or surgical care they seek in foreign countries, arrange for the transfer of medical records to the international providers, including the therapeutic recommendations of the domestic physicians, schedule procedures once the patient is agreeable with the proposal, arrange for visas and travel documents, book airplane flights and hotels, and in some cases, provide a representative in the host nation to assist with transfers and translation. Depending on the nature of the surgery, a recovery program may also be arranged, which may include necessary postoperative therapy or a vacation at a resort. The "surgeon and safari" program in South Africa offers patients the opportunity to recover in "authentic bush styled accommodations."[13]

Risks in Medical Tourism

Although these medical tours may sound enchanting on the surface, they are inappropriate or even impossible for most patients recovering from major surgery, including aesthetic surgery.

- There are major risks associated with traveling long distances before and after surgery, including venous thromboembolism and pulmonary embolism, dehydration, fatigue, pain, and disorientation.
- There is also no possibility of any preoperative face-to-face visit with the surgeon to establish a doctor-patient relationship, and no ability to directly consult with the surgeon postoperatively if a problem should occur after returning home.
- The sanitary conditions in some developing countries increase the risk of infections, including some that are rare in the United States, such as malaria, tuberculosis, and dysentery, as well as more common infectious diseases, which can be catastrophic in the postoperative patient.
- Language barriers can dramatically interfere with the quality of care because, even if the surgeon speaks English, the anesthetist, nurses, and aides often cannot, and they are responsible for much of the care.
- Similarly, even if the surgeon has received proper education and training, the quality of the preoperative and postoperative care largely depends on nurses and others who may have little or no education, training, or certification.
- It is difficult enough to identify the best surgeons in the United States, much less in a foreign country with differing processes for board certification and little or no information available about practitioner competence, success rates, deaths, and reputation.
- In most foreign countries, there is no ability to file a grievance if something goes wrong, either with the hospital or with the surgeon and, even if it is possible, it is impractical to pursue a complaint from thousands of miles away. The lack of malpractice insurance in foreign nations is partly responsible for the lower costs of care.
- If complications develop after returning home, it can be difficult to obtain care from the local physicians and hospitals, because they would automatically assume all the liability for a bad outcome even though they are not responsible for the cause of the complication, and received no reimbursement for the original care.
- The costs of care for such complications can be significant, and would quickly eliminate any savings realized from the original procedure.
- Traveling abroad to obtain experimental procedures or treatments increases the risks of unproved and potentially dangerous therapies, and using unapproved drugs or devices can lead to major complications, including

death, or becoming a victim of medical fraud and scams.

There are no large studies of the incidence of surgical complications and mortality comparing surgical care received abroad with that obtained in the United States, but anecdotal reports indicate that major complications are more commonly seen by American and British surgeons in patients who traveled abroad for care, and this is not unexpected in light of the numerous additional risks of medical tourism compared with care at home.

THE IMPACT OF INTERNATIONAL ACCREDITATION ON MEDICAL TOURISM

The outreach of the American accreditation agencies into international accreditation provides the potential of increasing patient safety for those who choose to travel abroad. Choosing hospitals and ambulatory surgery facilities that are accredited by AAAASF-I, JCI, or AAAHC International would reduce some of the many increased risks of medical tourism. Some would argue that these programs thereby encourage medical tourism, even although most increased risks are not minimized by accreditation. The motives for patients to seek surgical and dental care abroad are such that this medical travel will occur whether there is accreditation of facilities or not. The increase in accreditation does provide for increased patient safety and quality care for foreign patients as well as patients in those countries. It stimulates an increase in the quality of training for staff members, and higher standards for sanitation, medication, anesthesia, physical plants, and so forth. It also encourages the facilities that are not accredited to improve so that they may qualify for accreditation.

Traveling abroad for medical and surgical care has always existed, and it will continue to grow, for many reasons. Changes in medical coverage that may occur under health care reform in the United States may slow that growth, but medical tourism for aesthetic surgery will continue to grow for economic reasons. Rather than trying to stop this growth, improving the quality of care delivered is more realistic, and more beneficial.

SUMMARY

The growth of mandatory accreditation for ambulatory surgical facilities in the United States has been driven by:

a. the recognition by states that external oversight is required to ensure patient safety and quality

care in these centers where no standards previously existed and

b. the requirements of the commercial insurers that facilities be accredited, certified by Medicare, or licensed by the states to receive reimbursement for facility fees. As American accrediting organizations have begun international outreach efforts as a part of the general international movement in all aspects of American medicine, the growth of international accreditation has been driven by increasing demand for patient safety and quality care in all countries, and by the growth of medical tourism, with the marketing advantages of having an American accreditation.

REFERENCES

1. Code of Federal Regulations, Title 42, Chapter IV, Subchapter B, Part 416, Subpart B.
2. Federal Register, Vol. 61, Number 245, December 19, 1996.
3. Medical Group Management Association. ASC performance survey: 2009 report based on 2008 data. Washington, DC: MGMA; 2009.
4. California Business and Professions Code, Section 2216.
5. Iverson RE, Lynch DJ, the ASPS Task Force on Patient Safety in Officebased Surgery Facilities. Patient safety in office-based surgery facilities: II. Patient selection. Plast Reconstr Surg 2002;110(7): 1785–90.
6. Iverson RE, the ASPS Task Force on Patient Safety in Office-based Surgery Facilities. Patient safety in office-based surgery facilities: I. Procedures in the office-based surgery setting. Plast Reconstr Surg 2002;110(5):1337–42.
7. Byrd SH, Barton FE, Orenstein HH, et al. Safety and efficacy in an accredited outpatient plastic surgery facility: a review of 5316 consecutive cases. Plast Reconstr Surg 2003;112(2):636–41.
8. Keyes GR, Singer R, Iverson RE, et al. Analysis of outpatient surgery center safety using an Internet-based quality improvement and peer review program. Plast Reconstr Surg 2004;113(6):1760–70.
9. American Society of Plastic Surgeons bylaws, Article XV.
10. American Society for Aesthetic Plastic Surgery bylaws, Article XI.
11. Jones, DM. Global Economic Integration Drives Multinational Demand for Better Health Care. http://www.partners.org/Assets/Documents/International/Partners_Timeline_0309.pd; p. 4.
12. Kher U. Outsourcing your heart. Time 2006;167: 44–7.
13. Medical tourism: need surgery, will travel. CBC News Online, June 18, 2004.

Index

Note: Page numbers of article titles are in **boldface** type.

A

Accrediting organizations, national, 494
Aeronautic industry, checklists started in, 475–476
    lessons of, extended to health care, 476–477
Airway crisis, in airway management in outpatient setting, 412
Airway examination, elements of, 407
Airway management, in outpatient setting, **405–417**
    airway crisis and, 412
    airway obstruction and, 411–412
    aspiration and, 410–411
    history and physical examination for, 406–410
    intraoperative, complications of, 410
    laryngospasm and, 411
    operating room fire and, 412–415
    postoperative management in, 415
    preoperative planning for, 405–415
    staff and equipment for, 405–406
    ventilatory depression during sedation, 410
Airway obstruction, and airway management in outpatient setting, 411–412
Alcohol use, wound healing and, 442–443
American Association for Accreditation of Ambulatory Surgery Facilities, Inc., 465–466
    analysis of sequelae, 467
    data collection, 466
    data on rates of infection in outpatient surgery and, 440–441
    peer review, 466–467
    plastic surgery data, prevention of, 390–394
        risk assessment for, 390, 392
        September 2012, 390, 391–392
    sequelae types, 467–471
Anesthesia, effect of, on thermoregulation, 430, 431, 433
    for in-office endoscopy, 422–423
    local, and conscious sedation, in office-based surgical and procedural facility, **383–388**
Antibiotics, to reduce surgical site infections, 443–444
Antihistamines, in prevention of postoperative nausea and vomiting, 450
Aspiration, and airway management in outpatient setting, 410–411

B

Benzodiazepine, plus opioid, for in-office endoscopy, 422

Bleeding, as complication of endoscopy, 425
Blood glucose control, wound healing and, 443

C

Caprini Risk Assessment model (2010), deep venous thrombosis, 393, 394
Cardiopulmonary complications of endoscopy, 425
Chemoprophylaxis, of deep vein thrombosis, in plastic surgery, **399–404**
Children's Hospital Boston pediatric surgical safety checklist, 484, 485
Chlorhexadine shower, preoperative, to reduce infection, 445
Cholinergic antagonists, in prevention of postoperative nausea and vomiting, 450
Coagulation cascade, 400, 401
Colonoscopy, complications of, 425–426

D

Deep venous thrombosis, **389–398**
    chemoprophylaxis, agents for, 401–403
        dosing and timing for, 403
        in plastic surgery, **399–404**
    diagnosis of, 395–396
    discussion of, 396
    increased bleeding in, risk factors for, 394
    postoperative management in, 394
    prophylaxis regime, 394
    thrombus formation in, 400–401
    treatment of, 396
Dopamine, in prevention of postoperative nausea and vomiting, 449–450

E

Endoscopy, bleeding as complication of, 425
    cardiopulmonary complications of, 425
    complications in, 423–424
        unrelated to procedure, 424–426
    in-office, anesthesia for, 422–423
        benzodiazepines plus opioid for, 422
        documentation of, 426
        informed consent for, 422
        monitoring during, 423
        personnel for, 420–421
        postprocedure procedures in, 423
        preprocedure evaluation for, 421–422

plasticsurgery.theclinics.com

Printed and bound by CPI Group (UK) Ltd, Croydon, CR0 4YY

03/10/2024

01040346-0012